Colour **Aids**

Endocrinology

Peter H. Wise PhD FRCP FRACP
Consultant Physician, Department of Endocrinology,
Charing Cross Hospital, London, UK

Churchill Livingstone

EDINBURGH LONDON MELBOURNE AND NEW YORK 1986

Acknowledgements

The author appreciates the photographic contributions of Alison McCartney, Herbert Barrie, Ian Buttfield, Ilya Kovar, James McIvor, Tim Leonard, Julia Polak and John Lynn, and the generous help of the Department of Medical Illustration, Charing Cross & Westminster Medical School. Mrs Jaki Fagan was responsible for the painstaking and meticulous typing and setting out of the text.

P.H.W.

London, 1986

Contents

1 | Thyroid Deficiency

Neonatal hypothyroidism

Occurrence
Incidence approximately 1 : 5000 births.

**Aetiology/
Pathogenesis**
Agenesis or ectopic thyroid, maternal administration of excessive anti-thyroid drugs, congenital TSH deficiency, iodine deficiency.

**Clinical
features**
Hypotonia, coarse features, abdominal distension, occasional goitre.

Diagnosis
Absent distal femoral and proximal tibial epiphyses, low serum T4, elevated TSH (except in TSH deficiency).

Prevention
Avoidance of excessive anti-thyroid drugs in pregnancy, iodine prophylaxis in endemic areas, early diagnosis by neonatal screening.

Treatment
T4, initially 10 μg/kg daily, titrating to normalise serum TSH.

Complications
Untreated. Mental retardation, growth failure.
Treated. Overdosage leads to premature epiphyseal fusion of long bones (short stature) and cranial synostosis (mental retardation).

Juvenile hypothyroidism

**Occurrence
Aetiology/
Pathogenesis**
Prevalence approximately 1 : 1500 under age 20. As for adult hypothyroidism.

**Clinical
features**
Short stature, mental slowing (reversible), coarse skin, bradycardia, anaemia.

Diagnosis
As for adult hypothyroidism.
Radiology of hands shows delayed bone age.

Treatment
T4, 2−4 μg/kg per day, titrated to suppress TSH into normal range.

Complications
Untreated. Permanent short stature and mental retardation.
Treated. As for neonatal hypothyroidism.

THYROID DISORDERS

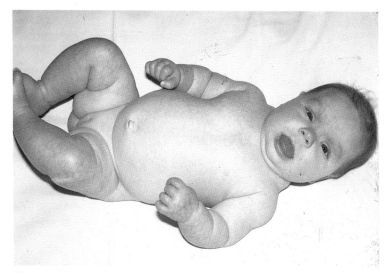

Fig. 1 Neonatal hypothyroidism: note large tongue and coarse features. Biochemical diagnosis achieved through routine neonatal screening.

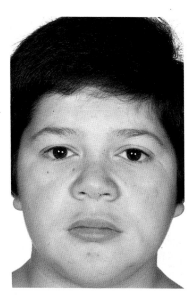

Fig. 2a Juvenile hypothyroidism in boy aged 16: coarse features, periorbital puffiness and sallow complexion. Height 150 cm.

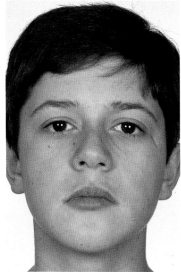

Fig 2b The same patient 12 months after treatment. Restoration of normal growth velocity.

2 | Adult Hypothyroidism
(Including Hashimoto's Disease)

Occurrence Prevalence approximately 1 : 150 over age 20.

Aetiology/ Pathogenesis

a. Autoimmune destructive lesion affecting follicular cell, occasionally blocking antibody to TSH receptor, or spontaneous transition from hyperthyroidism: associated with other disorders (see pp. 3, 9, 15, 33, 41, 93, 101) and with HLA-B8, DR3 and DR4.
b. Familial defect of hormone biosynthesis: hypothyroidism often precipitated by iodide or lithium.
c. Isolated TSH deficiency or pan-hypopituitarism (with or without tumour).
d. Thyroid hormone receptor insensitivity.
e. Following radioiodine, anti-thyroid drug excess, lithium or thyroid surgery.

Clinical features Occasionally absent. Subtle development of lethargy and malaise. Later coarse features, bradycardia, delayed reflex relaxation, cardiomyopathy, pericardial (and other serous) effusions, menorrhagia, dry thick skin, cerebellar ataxia and anaemia. Goitre sometimes present in (a), almost invariable in (b) and occasionally in (d).

Diagnosis Serum T4 low or low-normal. In groups (a), (b), (d) and (e), serum TSH elevated. Thyroid antibodies detectable in (a). High titre and firm goitre identifies Hashimoto's disease. Isotope uptake reduced (except (b) and (d)).

Prevention Life-long annual review of previously hyperthyroid cases, irrespective of therapy.

Treatment T4 50–200 μg/day, titrated to normalise serum TSH.

Complications *Untreated.* Depression and psychosis, proneness to hypothermia leading to stupor, coma and death (myxoedema coma), especially in the elderly. *Treated.* Excessive or rapid replacement of T4 may induce cardiac failure and precipitate angina or myocardial infarction.

THYROID DISORDERS

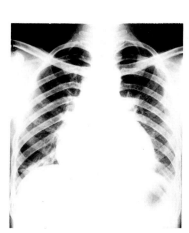

Fig. 3 Pericardial effusion in hypothyroidism (cardiothoracic ratio 0.7:1). Effusion confirmed by echocardiography.

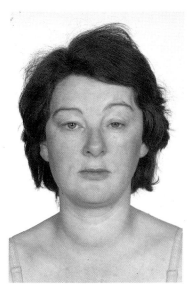

Fig. 4 Hypothyroidism and goitre due to lithium therapy. Patient had family history of autoimmune thyroid disease.

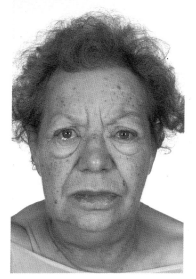

Fig. 5a Hypothyroidism presenting with lethargy, ataxia and confusion.

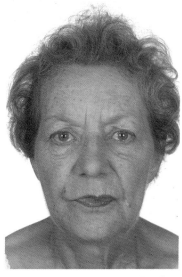

Fig. 5b Same patient 4 months after commencing therapy: total physical and neuropsychiatric recovery.

3 | Non-Toxic Goitre (Diffuse and Nodular)

Occurrence

Prevalence ranges from 1:100 to 1:3 in high and very low iodine intake areas respectively.

Aetiology/ Pathogenesis

a. Iodine deficiency: particularly common in hilly or mountainous areas (endemic goitre), sometimes associated with juvenile mental retardation (endemic goitrous cretinism).
b. Physiological: self-limiting in neonates, puberty and pregnancy.
c. Autoimmune thyroiditis (Hashimoto's disease).
d. Familial biosynthetic defects.
e. Drugs: lithium, vitamin A, phenylbutazone, thiocyanates, iodine and iodides (usually superimposed on biosynthetic defect).
f. Rarely carcinoma.

Clinical features

Symmetrical or mildly asymmetrical goitre, dysphagia or dyspnoea if retrosternal or large.

Diagnosis

History identifies iodine deficiency and drug effects. Thyroid antibody titre elevated in (c). Low salivary-to-plasma iodide ratio identifies trapping defect. Perchlorate discharge of pretrapped iodide confirms organification defect. Isotope or ultrasound scan defines multinodularity. Serum T4 and T3 to identify associated hyperthyroidism or hypothyroidism.

Treatment

T4 (100–200 µg) or T3 (60–100 µg) daily suppresses diffuse goitres especially in younger patients. Hashimoto's disease and multinodular goitre less responsive. Surgery for large or retrosternal goitres.

Complications

Untreated. Mediastinal compression if retrosternal, especially with haemorrhage into degenerating nodules.
Treated. Exogenous T4 or T3 may supplement autonomous T4 or T3 production (iatrogenic hyperthyroidism).

THYROID DISORDERS

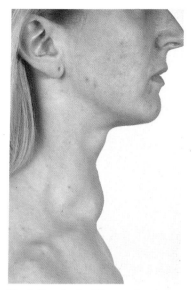

Fig. 6 Non-toxic diffuse goitre due to familial organification defect. Total resolution with T4 therapy.

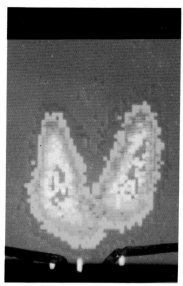

Fig. 7 ^{99m}Tc scan of same patient showing diffuse goitre: 30 min isotope uptake 8% (normal < 3.5%).

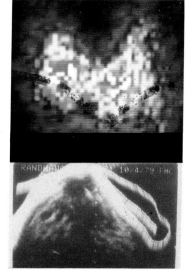

Fig. 8 ^{99m}Tc scan of MNG (above). Lower frame reveals cystic (dark) areas in right lobe using ultrasound.

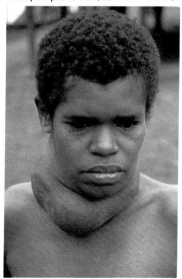

Fig. 9 Endemic goitre in a New Guinea native.

4 | Localised Thyroid Nodule
(Including Carcinoma)

Occurrence

Prevalence less than 1 : 100 over age 20.

**Aetiology/
Pathogenesis**

a. Thyroid cyst, with or without haemorrhage.
b. Colloid nodule.
c. True adenoma.
d. Malignant papillary, follicular, anaplastic or
   medullary thyroid (C-cell) carcinoma.
   Lymphoma.

**Clinical
features**

Incidental finding of nodule. Sudden evolution
with pain suggests haemorrhage into cyst.
Hoarseness and dysphagia suggest malignancy.
Lymphadenopathy and systemic symptoms in
metastatic malignancy. Medullary thyroid
carcinoma sometimes familial, in association with
phaeochromocytoma and hyperparathyroidism.
MEA type II and III (see p. 99): metastatic disease
often associated with ectopic ACTH (see p. 95)
syndrome and diarrhoea. Hyperthyroidism
occasionally in solitary hyperfunctioning nodules
(see p. 13).

Diagnosis

Isotope scan identifies tissue avidity: 'hot' less
likely malignant than 'cold' nodules. Thin needle
aspiration cytology 95% reliable in separating
benign from malignant lesions. Ultrasound
identifies cystic lesions. Serum calcitonin
represents tissue marker for C-cell tumours.
Serum thyroglobulin level indicates extent of
malignant metastases in non-C-cell tumours.
Serum T4 and T3 levels identify hyperthyroidism.

Treatment

Cysts have 50% recurrence after aspiration.
Confirmed benign lesions require treatment only
if cosmetic. Lymphoma usually responsive to
radiotherapy/chemotherapy. Confirmed papillary
or follicular carcinoma treated by total
thyroidectomy followed by radioiodine ablation
of demonstrable iodine-avid metastases. C-cell
tumours may justify familial screening.

THYROID DISORDERS

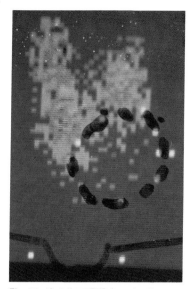

Fig. 10 'Cold' nodule (marked) on isotope scan in patient presenting with solitary swelling. Aspiration cytology confirmed papillary carcinoma.

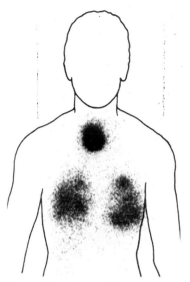

Fig. 11 Whole-body I^{131} scan following partial thyroidectomy for carcinoma thyroid. Scan reveals residual thyroid uptake and 'pneumogram' of multiple pulmonary metastases.

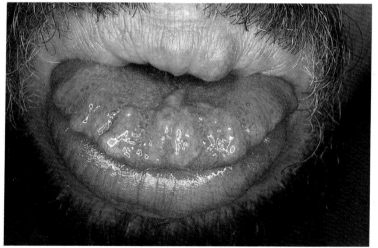

Fig. 12 Nodular fibromas on lip and tongue in patient with medullary thyroid carcinoma. Patient also had hypertension due to pheochromocytoma (Sipple's syndrome).

5 | Toxic Diffuse Goitre
(Graves' Disease) (1)

Occurrence

Prevalence 1:200 over age 20; F : M, 2 : 1.

Aetiology/ Pathogenesis

Abnormal (i.e. non-TSH) thyroid stimulators which are antibodies (immunoglobulins) to TSH-receptors. Predisposing factors: HLA-B8, DR3 and DR4. Often associated with other familial organ-specific autoimmune disorders (see pp. 3, 15, 33, 41, 93, 101). Some cases precipitated by excess iodide (Jod-Basedow). Transient hyperthyroidism, especially post-partum, may represent a variant.

Clinical features

Occasionally absent. Tachycardia, sweating, tremor, anxiety and lid lag and retraction are due to adrenergic potentiation. Weight loss, heat intolerance, tiredness and weakness (myopathy) secondary to hypermetabolism. Goitre is usually present. Proptosis (ophthalmopathy) with diplopia (ocular myopathy) and chemosis (conjunctival oedema), thyroid acropachy (pseudoclubbing) and pretibial myxoedema (dermopathy) unrelated to hormone excess, and represent infiltrative processes due to different immunoglobulins.

Diagnosis

Serum T4 and T3 high or high-normal. Serum T3 alone occasionally raised (T3-toxicosis). Serum TSH suppressed, and non-responsive to 200 µg i.v. TRH. Thyroid scan shows diffuse goitre with increased isotopic (I^{131} or ^{99m}Tc) uptake.

Treatment

Beta-adrenergic blockade useful for symptomatic control. Anti-thyroid drugs (carbimazole, propylthiouracil) block organification of iodide and suppress immunoglobulins. Remission rate 50–70% after 12 months of therapy. Subtotal thyroidectomy for very large or retrosternal goitres or post-drug relapse (remission rate 80–90%). Radioactive iodine indicated in post-surgical relapse and primary treatment where transition to hypothyroidism is acceptable (remission rate 95–100%).

THYROID DISORDERS

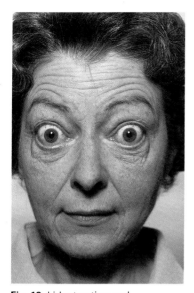

Fig. 13 Lid retraction and exophthalmos in patient with Graves' disease.

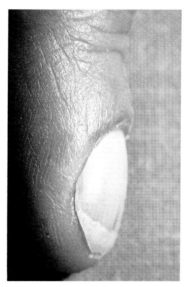

Fig. 14 Thyroid acropachy (pseudo-clubbing): nail-bed recession (onycholysis) also present.

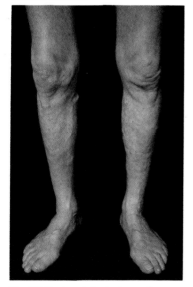

Fig. 15 Red nodular lesions of infiltrative dermopathy (pretibial myxoedema).

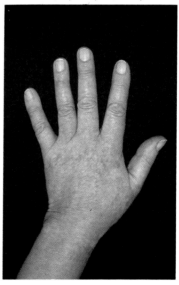

Fig. 16 Depigmentation (vitiligo) of hand in patient with Graves' disease.

5	# Toxic Diffuse Goitre **(Graves' Disease) (2)**
Treatment (cont)	Ophthalmopathy treated by tarsorrhaphy, or if progressive, by high dose corticosteroids and occasionally orbital decompression.
Complications	*Untreated*. Cardiomyopathy in severe or prolonged disease. Hyperthyroid crisis (storm) often precipitated by intercurrent illness; hyperpyrexia, confusion and adrenergic features, fatal if untreated. Therapy includes rehydration, beta blockade, intravenous iodide and high dose anti-thyroid drugs. *Treated*. Hypothyroidism in 3−5% drug-treated, 15−20% surgical and 20−50% radioiodine-treated cases. Risk of hypoparathyroidism and recurrent laryngeal nerve damage after surgery.
6	# Sub-acute Thyroiditis **(de Quervain's disease)**
Occurrence	Unknown: many mild cases probably undiagnosed.
Aetiology/ Pathogenesis	Some cases may be virally induced. Cycle of inflammation with acute hormonal discharge, sometimes followed by a temporary and variable degree of hypothyroidism, but with eventual return to euthyroidism in 95% of patients.
Clinical features	Simulates Graves' disease, but without ophthalmopathy or dermopathy. Thyroid often painful.
Diagnosis	As for Graves' disease, but isotopic uptake and scan totally suppressed.
Treatment	Aspirin and occasionally corticosteroids.
Complications	Hypothyroidism permanent in 3−5% of cases.

THYROID DISORDERS

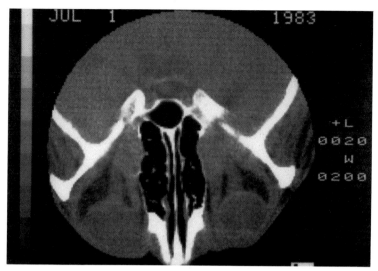

Fig. 17 CT scan of orbits in thyroid ophthalmopathy: marked swelling of extraocular muscles, especially adjacent to nasal cavity (medial rectus).

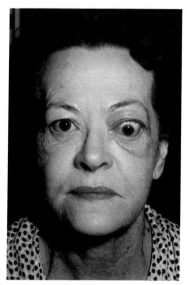

Fig. 18 Asymmetric thyroid ophthalmopathy simulating retro-orbital tumour: the patient was biochemically thyrotoxic.

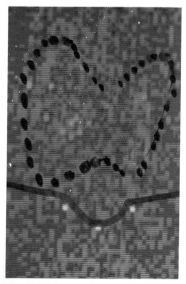

Fig. 19 Subacute thyroiditis: patient thyrotoxic but scan image 'suppressed' (palpable gland outline marked).

7 | Toxic Nodular Goitre

Occurrence

Prevalence approximately 1:500 over age 20.

Aetiology/ Pathogenesis

a. *Autonomous hyperfunctioning nodule (AFN).* true adenoma or single regenerating nodule.
b. *Multinodular toxic goitre (MTG).* Multifocal regenerating nodules in a long-standing previously non-toxic gland. Occasionally hyperthyroidism is precipitated by iodide excess (drugs, contrast media).

Clinical features

Solitary palpable nodule; multinodular goitre, sometimes retrosternal and with occasional upper mediastinal compression (dysphagia, dyspnoea, hoarseness). Clinical features of hypermetabolism and adrenergic hyperfunction (see p. 9), but without ophthalmopathy. Cardiomyopathy is common, especially with atrial fibrillation.

Diagnosis

Biochemical diagnosis as for toxic diffuse goitre (see p. 9), but isotopic scan shows either (a) single hyperfunctioning nodule exceeding 2 cm diameter suppressing uptake in remainder of gland, or (b) multifocal isotopic aggregation.

Treatment

a. *AFN.* Re-scan after TSH 10 units i.m. to identify potential recruitment of suppressed thyroid, then either nodule excision or radioiodine therapy.
b. *MTG.* Large dose radioiodine therapy (may require multiple doses), or subtotal thyroidectomy if goitre very large or retrosternal.

Complications

Untreated. Atrial fibrillation with systemic embolism. Refractory cardiac failure.
Treated. Hypothyroidism incidence <5% with radioiodine therapy.

THYROID DISORDERS

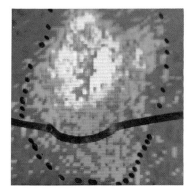

Fig. 20 Isotope scan of large toxic nodular goitre with retrosternal extension inducing marked dysphagia (sternoclavicular region and gland outline marked).

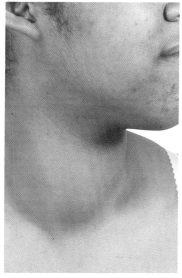

Fig. 21 Hyperthyroidism in a 20-year-old girl with palpable right lobe nodule.

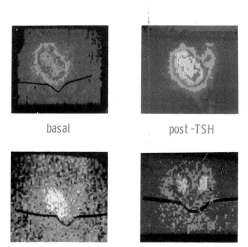

basal

post-TSH

4 months post treatment   15 months post treatment

Fig. 22 Scan sequence of patient in Figure 21, showing initial autonomous hyperfunctioning nodule, recruitment of previously suppressed left lobe after TSH, and the response to ablative radioiodine at 4 and 15 month follow-up.

Diabetes Mellitus (1)

Occurrence

Prevalence 0.5–2 : 100, but in some ethnic groups up to 20 : 100 (Australian Aboriginals, Pima Indians).

Aetiology/ Pathogenesis

Type I (insulin-dependent). Association with HLA-B8, DR3, DR4 and with other familial thyrogastric autoimmune disorders (see pp. 3, 9, 33, 41, 93, 101). All cases have beta-cell damage, possibly virus-precipitated autoimmune destruction.
Type II (non-insulin-dependent). Strong familial beta-cell and peripheral tissue metabolic defect. Hyperglycaemia often precipitated by stress, obesity or drugs (diuretics, corticosteroids).
Secondary. Due to pancreatitis or carcinoma, haemochromatosis and other endocrinopathies (acromegaly, Cushing's syndrome, glucagonoma).

Clinical features

Type I. Usually acute onset polyuria, polydipsia and weight loss leading to coma if undiagnosed. Most common under age 50.
Type II. Many cases asymptomatic, especially in over-50 age group. Usually insidious polyuria and polydipsia. Infections may both result from, and induce, hyperglycaemia.
Secondary. Clinical features of underlying disorder; polyuria and polydipsia variable in onset and severity.

Diagnosis

Glycosuria in most cases; ketonuria is almost invariable in type I diabetes. Random blood glucose > 12 mmol/l is diagnostic and glucose tolerance test is rarely necessary. Islet-cell antibodies present in more than 50% of type I cases, decreasing over subsequent five years.

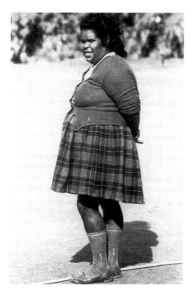

Fig. 23 Obesity: a major determinant of the 15–20% diabetes prevalence in Australian Aboriginals.

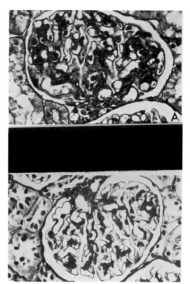

Fig. 24 Diabetic microangiopathy: basement membrane thickening in diabetic renal glomerulus (above), normal glomerulus below.

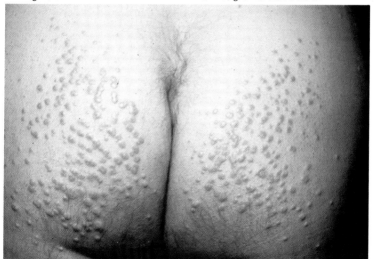

Fig. 25 Eruptive xanthomatosis in a newly diagnosed diabetic. Lesions disappeared within 6 weeks of achieving normoglycaemia.

Treatment

In all cases, a diet low in fat and high in fibre, with constant calories from day to day and also within-day distribution.

Type I. Insulin is invariably necessary. Optimum control requires 2–4 injections daily, or continuous subcutaneous or intraperitoneal pump infusion, ideally monitored by home blood glucose measurement to maintain normoglycaemia.

Type II. Calorie restriction alone is effective in 50% of cases; remaining patients are controllable by a sulphonylurea and/or biguanide drug, and only rarely require insulin, except with dietary non-compliance. Monitoring by urine (or blood) glucose measurement is essential and increased exercise is beneficial in all cases.

Complications

Metabolic

1. *Hypoglycaemia.* Transient faintness, hunger, tremor and ultimately confusion and coma are secondary to insulin excess, omission of food or inappropriate exercise.

2. *Ketoacidosis (DKA).* Usually illness-induced severe hyperglycaemia and glycosuria, ketonaemia and ketonuria lead to dehydration, vomiting and progressive drowsiness and coma. Treatment is with insulin infusion and rehydration. Mortality should be less than 5%.

3. *Hyperosmolar coma.* Gross hyperglycaemia and dehydration without ketoacidosis, often in type II diabetes. Treatment by rehydration and low dose insulin. Mortality approximately 30%.

4. *Lactic acidosis.* Precipitated by acute ischaemia, e.g. myocardial infarction, mostly in the presence of renal or hepatic disease, interfering with lactate clearance. Mortality exceeds 80%.

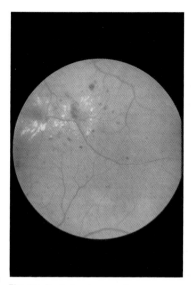

Fig. 26 Early background retinopathy in a diabetic of 15 years duration: dot and blot haemorrhages and exudates.

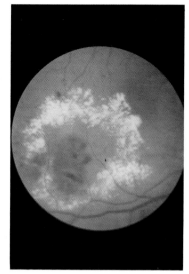

Fig. 27 Diabetic maculopathy: central visual field defect clinically documented.

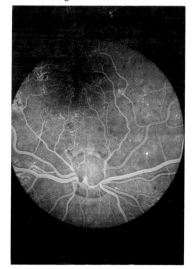

Fig. 28 Fluorescein angiogram showing microaneurysms (white dots): fundus appeared normal to conventional retinoscopy.

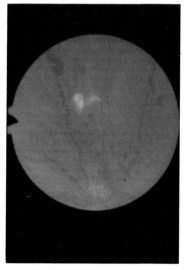

Fig. 29 Proliferative retinopathy: marked neovascularisation and venular dilatation.

Complications
(cont)

Metabolic (cont)
5. *Hyperlipidaemia.* Hypertriglyceridaemia secondary to prolonged poor control; clinically manifest by reversible eruptive xanthomatosis.
6. *Arteriosclerosis.* Accelerated development in diabetes especially involving cerebral, coronary, and lower limb vessels, resulting in cerebrovascular lesions, myocardial ischaemia and intermittent claudication respectively.

Ocular
1. *Visual blurring.* Due to reversible hyperglycaemic osmotic lens changes.
2. *Cataract.* Early onset (central) lesion or accelerated senile (peripheral) lens changes.
3. *Extraocular muscle paralysis.* Secondary to transient mononeuritis of 3rd, 4th, or 6th cranial nerves.
4. *Retinopathy.* Microangiopathic damage leading to increased capillary permeability, haemorrhage and vascular occlusion and related to diabetic control and duration. *Background retinopathy (BR).* asymptomatic haemorrhage and exudate; visual field impairment only if at macula (maculopathy). *Proliferative retinopathy (PR).* neovascularisation secondary to retinal ischaemia and resulting in pre-retinal vitreous haemorrhage, eventually with fibrotic traction detachment of the retina and blindness. *Macular oedema*: central visual field loss due to capillary hyperpermeability. BR and PR are treatable by early recognition and laser photocoagulation. Advanced cases are sometimes amenable to vitrectomy.
5. *Rubeosis iridis.* Neovascularisation of iris with secondary haemorrhage.

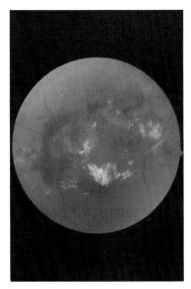

Fig. 30 Pre-retinal haemorrhage in proliferative retinopathy.

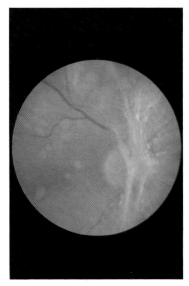

Fig. 31 Retinitis proliferans. Fibrous contraction resulted in retinal detachment 6 months later.

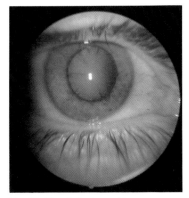

Fig. 32 'Senile' cataract in a 50-year-old diabetic: inwardly radiating spicules.

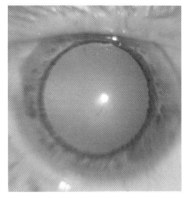

Fig. 33 Early posterior subcapsular cataract (below light reflex) in a 28-year-old diabetic of 15 years duration

Complications
(cont)

Renal
1. *Pyelonephritis.* Increased susceptibility.
2. *Diabetic nephropathy.* Microangiopathic renal glomerular damage, related to control and duration of diabetes, resulting in proteinuria and later hypoproteinaemia, oedema, hypertension and renal failure. Haemodialysis and transplantation sometimes required. Control of hypertension and possibly of hyperglycaemia improves survival.
3. *Necrotising papillitis.* Sequestration of a renal papilla, secondary to diabetic vascular disease, infection and/or analgesics, resulting in loin pain and/or urinary tract obstruction.

Neurological
1. *Mononeuritis.* Usually a reversible lesion affecting peripheral motor, sensory or cranial nerves, often at the onset of diabetes.
2. *Symmetrical sensorimotor neuropathy.* Affecting dominantly the feet and predisposing to injury with subsequent infection; typical plantar ulceration; occasionally neuropathic arthropathy.
3. *Amyotrophy.* Symmetrical, painful proximal motor nerve root involvement, usually of the lower limbs; usually self-limiting.
4. *Autonomic neuropathy.* Postural hypotension, impotence, intestinal motility disorder and malabsorption; bladder dysfunction.

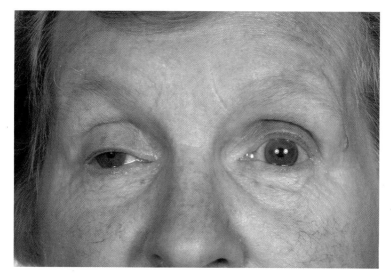

Fig. 34 Right 3rd nerve palsy (ptosis and abducted right eye) in newly diagnosed diabetic: reverted to normal within 3 months of achieving control.

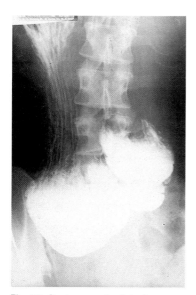

Fig. 35 Gastroparesis diabeticorum in a grossly unstable diabetic. Barium still in stomach at 8 hours.

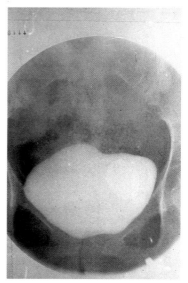

Fig. 36 Atonic neurogenic bladder. Patient (aged 23) suffered recurrent urinary tract infection.

Complications
(cont)

Skin
1. Increased risk of *staphylococcal sepsis and fungal infections*.
2. *Necrobiosis lipoidica diabeticorum*. Lesions of unknown aetiology manifest by a metabolic and microvascular component affecting arms, legs and occasionally face.
3. *Hypertrophy or atrophy of subcutaneous injection sites*. Usually seen only with use of unpurified insulins.
4. *Erythematous, bullous dermatitis* in association with glucagonoma syndrome.
5. *Allergic reactions*, especially to unpurified insulins.

The diabetic foot
Foot complications are responsible for most diabetes admissions. Peripheral neuropathy predisposes to undetected injury, with healing impaired by macro- and/or microvascular disease and superimposed infection. Ulceration develops and can proceed rapidly to gangrene, or to underlying bone involvement (osteoyelitis) in some cases. Amputation is often required.

Pregnancy
The increased incidence of toxaemia, hydramnios, prematurity, congenital abnormalities, and fetal macrosomia are all minimised by optimal diabetic control. Neonatal respiratory distress syndrome is less frequent with improved diabetic control and near-normal time of delivery.

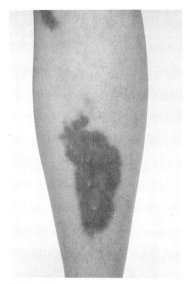

Fig. 37 Necrobiosis lipoidica in a 24-year-old girl.

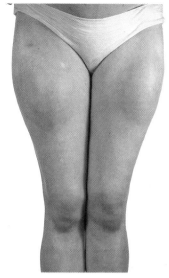

Fig. 38 Fat hypertrophy in a 20-year-old girl: resolution followed transfer to purified insulin.

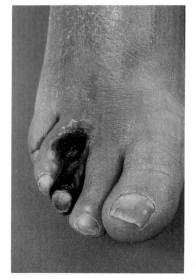

Fig. 39 Gangrene from self-pedicure. Diabetic neuropathy and absent pulses. Cellulitis present.

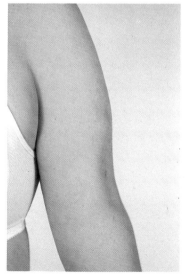

Fig. 40 Fat atrophy from use of unpurified (protamine zinc) insulin.

9 | Insulinoma

Occurrence

Rare.

**Aetiology/
Pathogenesis**

A tumour of beta cells of the islets of Langerhans: histology shows adenoma, or less frequently, carcinoma. Some cases appear to be associated with islet-cell hyperplasia, cause unknown.

**Clinical
features**

Spontaneous sweating, confusion, coma and occasionally convulsions, precipitated by fasting, exercise and occasionally alcohol. Episodes respond rapidly to oral or intravenous dextrose.

Diagnosis

The combination of low plasma glucose (<2 mmol/l) at the time of the episode, together with an inappropriately high plasma insulin (> 10 mU/l) at the time of hypoglycaemia is virtually diagnostic. Attempted induction of hypoglycaemia or prolonged fasting usually not required for diagnosis. It is important to exclude iatrogenic hypoglycaemia (sulphonylureas), alcohol-hypoglycaemia and hypopituitarism as other common causes of hypoglycaemia. Radiological localisation is by coeliac axis angiography, or by transhepatic venous sampling. Isotopic methods are usually unsatisfactory.

Treatment

Surgical excision of previously localised adenoma. 'Blind' subtotal pancreatectomy without previous identification is considered undesirable; repeat attempted localisation is ideally deferred for twelve months and medical therapy provided. Propranolol and diazoxide are of value in temporary medical treatment; streptozotocin is employed in metastatic malignant insulinoma.

Complications

Untreated. Organic brain syndrome and dementia, together with death from hypoglycaemia in undiagnosed cases.
Treated. Diabetes develops in 10% of operated cases.

CARBOHYDRATE DISORDERS

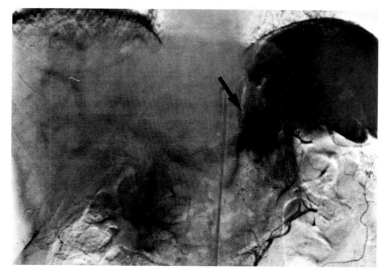

Fig. 41 Subtraction film of arteriogram in patient with spontaneous hypoglycaemia. Tumour blush (arrow) identifies large insulinoma in tail of pancreas.

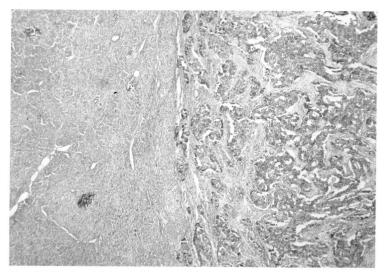

Fig. 42 Histology of same tumour stained for insulin (brown). Normal islet within normal pancreas on left; widespread staining within tumour on right.

10 | Non-secreting Hypothalamic-pituitary Tumours

Occurrence

True incidence unknown: uncommon.

Aetiology/ Pathogenesis

Suprasellar tumours. Craniopharyngioma—arises from Rathke's pouch rest cells, usually presenting in childhood. Arachnoid cysts, hamartomas (congenital malformation), pinealomas, astrocytomas, epidermoid tumours and meningiomas are less common.
Intrasellar tumours. Lesions mentioned above may secondarily involve the sella; pituitary adenoma is the most common primary intrasellar lesion, and may extend into the suprasellar region. Secondary (metastatic) tumours, especially from breast may occur.

Clinical features

Occasionally asymptomatic headache and vomiting from increased intracranial pressure due to aqueduct obstruction, or visual loss from involvement of optic chiasma, together with varying degrees of hypopituitarism (see p. 33), particularly growth failure in children and diabetes insipidus in adults.

Diagnosis

Lateral skull X-ray may show calcification in craniopharyngioma and meningioma or expanded pituitary fossa. CT scan reveals site of tumours or evidence of aqueduct obstruction. Endocrine assays are required to confirm the extent of endocrine deficiency, and serum prolactin to exclude functioning pituitary adenoma. Visual field assessments are essential to confirm or exclude chiasmal involvement.

Treatment

Most suprasellar tumors require surgery; some (craniopharyngioma) may be radio-sensitive. Endocrine replacement therapy is required where deficiencies are documented.

Complications

Untreated. Most lesions are progressive.
Treated. Surgery or radiotherapy may occasionally induce further endocrine deficiencies—immediate after surgery, and delayed after radiotherapy.

PITUITARY DISORDERS

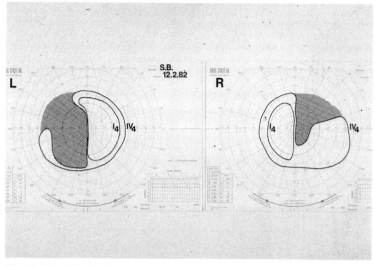

Fig. 43 Visual fields of patient with craniopharyngioma. Typical bitemporal defect using small, high-intensity object (I_4); asymmetrical chiasmal involvement disclosed using larger high intensity object (IV_4).

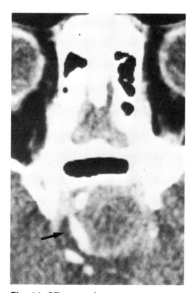

Fig. 44 CT scan of craniopharyngioma showing calcification (arrow) at rim of less dense tumour mass.

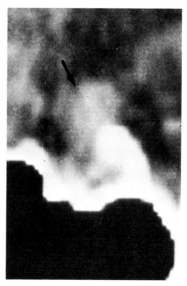

Fig. 45 CT scan of patient with diabetes insipidus and breast carcinoma: arrow shows metastatic hypothalamic deposit above normal pituitary fossa.

11 | Pituitary Prolactinoma

Occurrence | Unknown. Probably less than 1 : 2000.

Aetiology/ Pathogenesis | A benign tumour of prolactin-producing cells. Defective hypothalamic dopaminergic pathways possibly responsible. Pregnancy and exogenous oestrogen can promote growth of existing tumours.

Clinical features | Oligo- or amenorrhea, loss of libido and potency, infertility and galactorrhea. Occasionally, hirsutism or other evidence of benign androgen excess (acne, seborrhea) are present. Uncommonly, tumours expand to produce optic chiasmal compression, or other pituitary hormone deficiencies.

Diagnosis | Prolactinoma is the commonest cause of non-puerperal galactorrhea; phenothiazine and benzodiazepine drugs and other dopamine antagonists, hypothyroidism, chronic self-stimulation and rare malignancies (ectopic hormone production) require exclusion. Serum prolactin elevated. Skull X-rays reveal sella enlargement, or destruction in larger tumours. CT scan displays most small intrasellar microadenomas. Thyroid, growth hormone and adrenal function are often normal.

Treatment | Not all cases require therapy. Infertility and galactorrhea usually respond to dopamine agonists (bromocriptine 2.5–10 mg daily, or equivalent doses of lisuride or pergolide), and tumours mostly reduce in size. Subsequent therapy with either megavoltage radiotherapy (40–50 Gy) or trans-sphenoidal selective excision in some cases.

Complications | *Untreated*. Natural history of expansion is not known but probably slow. Haemorrhage into, or infarction of, tumour causes hypopituitarism or spontaneous resolution (rarely).
Treated. Gastrointestinal intolerance to dopamine agonist drugs. Immediate (surgical) or delayed (radiotherapy) development of hypopituitarism occurs in 5–20% of cases. Recurrence of prolactinoma after surgery is occasionally seen.

PITUITARY DISORDERS

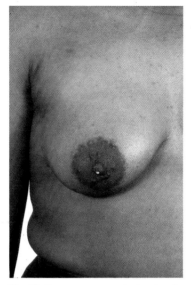

Fig. 46 Spontaneous galactorrhea in a patient with a small prolactinoma.

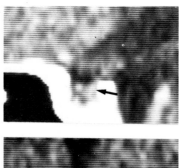

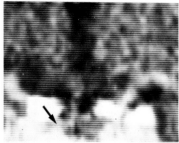

Fig. 47 CT scan appearance of 3 mm prolactinoma (arrow) in sagittal (upper) and coronal (lower) section.

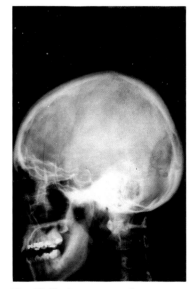

Fig. 48 Pituitary macroadenoma (serum prolactin 35 000 nmol/l): note double contour fossa floor denoting asymmetric tumour.

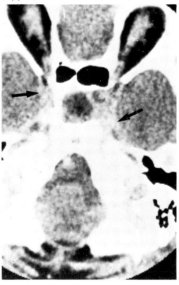

Fig. 49 CT scan of extrasellar tumour extension (arrows) of initially intrasellar prolactinoma.

12 | Acromegaly

Occurrence

Prevalence: approximately 1 : 40 000.

Aetiology/ Pathogenesis

A primary tumour of pituitary somatotrophs, leading to hypertrophy of all tissues and increased longitudinal growth if developing before epiphyseal fusion completed.

Clinical features

Gigantism if originating under age 20. Coarsening of all features, increased foot and hand size, excessive sweating and seborrhea, and headaches, lethargy and narcolepsy. Increased incidence of cutaneous papillomas and fibromas. Arthralgia and back pain due to bone deformity. Cardiomegaly and overt cardiomyopathy occur in severe prolonged cases. Hypertension and diabetes are common. Evidence of extrasellar extension (chiasmal compression) and hypopituitarism with larger tumours.

Diagnosis

Serum growth hormone levels fail to suppress to below 2 mU/l during glucose tolerance test. Somatomedin-C levels elevated. Skull X-ray may show enlarged sella, mandible and frontal sinuses. Other specific tests of pituitary function may reveal evidence of associated endocrine deficiencies (see p. 33). CT scan shows tumour size.

Treatment

Some cases respond to dopamine agonist therapy (e.g. bromocriptine up to 40 mg daily), occasionally with regression in tumour size. Preferable therapy is either external megavoltage irradiation or yttrium implantation (40–60% remission rate), or transphenoidal tumour removal (40–80% remission rate depending on size).

Complications

Untreated. Progressive disability, especially manifest by chiasmal compression, osteoarthritis and bone pain. Premature death from stroke, intractable cardiac failure or arrythmias. *Treated.* Gastrointestinal symptoms from dopamine agonist therapy. Early (surgery) or late (radiotherapy) hypopituitarism (10–50% over 10 years).

PITUITARY DISORDERS

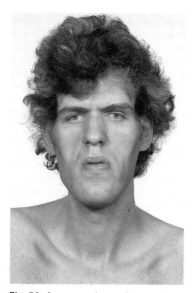

Fig. 50 Acromegaly: patient was entirely asymptomatic.

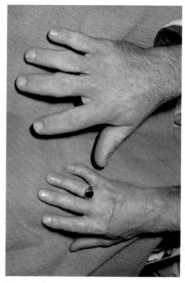

Fig. 51 Acromegalic compared with normal male hand.

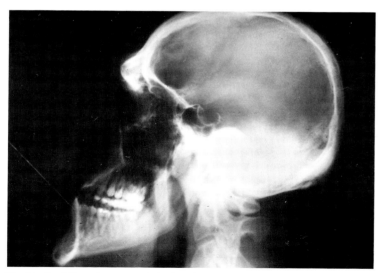

Fig. 52 Skull X-ray in acromegaly showing prominent frontal ridge, prognathism and expansion of pituitary fossa by tumour.

Occurrence

Prevalence: approximately 1 : 5000.

**Aetiology/
Pathogenesis**

Secondary to space-occupying benign or metastatic malignant tumours.
Vascular. Haemorrhage into pituitary adenoma; post-partum infarction (Sheehan's syndrome); carotid artery aneurysm.
Infiltration and granulomas. Histiocytosis, sarcoidosis, haemochromatosis.
Infections. Tuberculosis, post-meningitic.
Traumatic. Following head injury.
Iatrogenic. Following megavoltage radiotherapy or surgery.
Empty-sella syndrome. Primary or secondary to pituitary tumour infarction.
Idiopathic hypopituitarism. With or without associated familial thyrogastric autoimmune disorder (see pp. 3, 9, 15, 41, 93, 101).
Isolated pituitary hormone deficiency. Deficiency of hGH, TSH, LH/FSH, ACTH, ADH, possibly due to hypothalamic dysfunction.

**Clinical
features**

These depend on the underlying pathology. Even after vascular episode (e.g. post-partum infarction), clinical presentation may not appear for many years. Tiredness, depression, anaemia are common and non-specific. Other clinical features depend on the extent of endocrine deficiency including amenorrhoea, impotence, and signs and symptoms of hypothyroidism, together with generalised loss of body hair and hypotension. In childhood, short stature may be the presenting feature. Acute presentation is often precipitated by inter-current infection, trauma, surgery or anaesthesia resulting in hypopituitary crisis, with hypotension, hypothermia and collapse.

PITUITARY DISORDERS

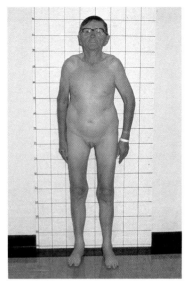

Fig. 53 55-year-old man with 'idiopathic' hypopituitarism: sister had pernicious anaemia. Note absent body hair and small genitalia.

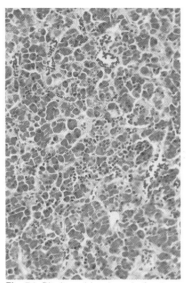

Fig. 54 Pituitary histology in fatal undiagnosed case of idiopathic hypopituitarism: note lymphocytic infiltrate.

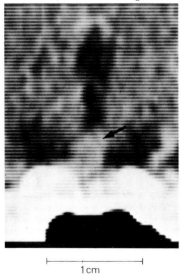

|—— 1 cm ——|

Fig. 55 High resolution CT scan of patient MM: diabetes insipidus and hypogonadism. Arrow shows pituitary stalk lesion: 3rd ventricle above.

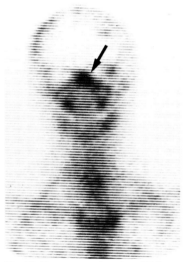

Fig. 56 Bone scan of patient MM showing pituitary 'hot' spot. Biopsy of a further rib lesion confirmed histiocytosis X.

13 | Hypopituitarism (2)

Diagnosis

Confirmation of endocrine deficiency as follows:
TSH. Low serum T4 and TSH: TSH response to TRH may differentiate hypothalamic (positive) from pituitary (negative) cause.
ACTH. Low urinary and plasma cortisol, with non-response of plasma cortisol to insulin-induced hypoglycaemia or CRF infusion. Retained cortisol response to synthetic ACTH.
LH/FSH. Low testosterone or oestradiol with low LH and FSH.
hGH. Failure of serum hGH to rise above 20 mU/l with strenuous exercise or insulin hypoglycaemia/arginine stimulation. hGH releasing hormone infusion may differentiate hypothalamic from pituitary causes.
ADH. Fluid deprivation fails to raise urine osmolality above 600 mmol/kg. Hypertonic saline infusion fails to stimulate diagnostic rise in serum AVP (ADH).
Skull radiology and CT scan are required to identify underlying pathology.

Treatment

Management of the underlying disease. Replacement therapy as appropriate with thyroxine 50–200 µg daily, hydrocortisone 10–30 mg daily, oestrogens or androgens especially in patients under age 50. Growth hormone (human or synthetic) therapy is indicated in dwarfism (see also p. 77). Desmopressin nasal spray in diabetes insipidus: occasionally chlorpropramide orally suffices in mild cases.

Complications

Untreated. Death frequent in undiagnosed cases from hypothermia and hypotension, usually precipitated by stress. Osteoporosis common where oestrogens/androgens not replaced.
Treated. Steroid crises due to inadequate steroid supplementation during stress periods.

PITUITARY DISORDERS

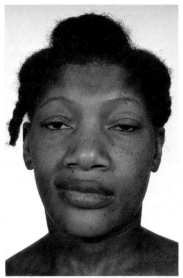

Fig. 57 Hypopituitarism presenting 15 years after post-partum haemorrhage.

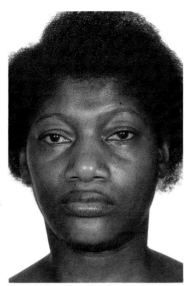

Fig. 58 Same patient 6 months after commencing hydrocortisone and thyroxine: restoration of skin texture and facial contours.

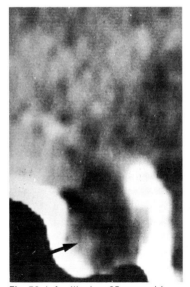

Fig. 59 Infertility in a 25-year-old girl: sagittal CT reconstruction shows mainly 'empty' sella (dark) with minimal pituitary tissue (arrow).

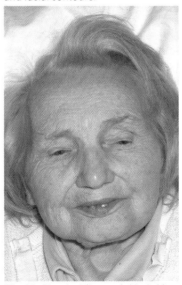

Fig. 60 Classical fine, wrinkled skin in elderly hypopituitary patient presenting with hypotension and hypothermia.

14 | Cushing's Syndrome (1)

Occurrence

Prevalence approximately 1 : 20 000.

**Aetiology/
Pathogenesis**

1. *Pituitary-dependent adrenal hyperplasia
(Cushing's disease).* ACTH-producing pituitary
macro- or microadenoma, possibly secondary to
hypothalamic CRF dysregulation.
2. *Adrenal tumour.* Unilateral autonomous
hyperfunctioning adenoma or carcinoma: cause
unknown, but occasionally associated with other
endocrine adenomas (pancreatic beta-cell,
parathyroid and/or pituitary adenoma—Wermer's
syndrome, see p. 99.
3. *Ectopic ACTH syndrome.* Bilateral adrenal
hyperplasia secondary to production of abnormal
ACTH or precursors from non-endocrine
malignant neoplasms, often bronchial oat-cell or
medullary thyroid (C-cell) carcinoma, (see p. 7).
4. *Iatrogenic Cushing's syndrome.* Excessive
administration of exogenous corticosteroids in
the course of treatment of inflammatory
disorders.

**Clinical
features**

Truncal obesity, with facial plethora,
hypertension, cutaneous striae, bruising,
osteoporosis, amenorrhoea and poor wound
healing; growth retardation in children. In most
cases mild hirsutism, but in adenoma patients
more striking and may be the presenting
symptom. Weakness is common but especially in
ectopic ACTH syndrome (due to associated
severe hypokalaemic myopathy) in which other
Cushingoid features are often lacking. Mild
pigmentation in (1), and in (3), especially
associated with C-cell tumours. Symptoms or
signs of expanding pituitary tumour in (1)
uncommon.

ADRENAL DISORDERS

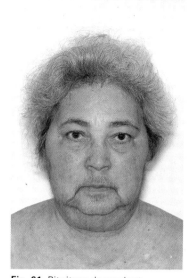

Fig. 61 Pituitary-dependent Cushing's disease: marked hirsutism, facial plethora and supraclavicular fat pads.

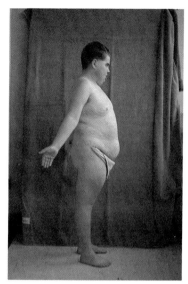

Fig. 62 Juvenile Cushing's disease: gross truncal obesity, striae and short stature.

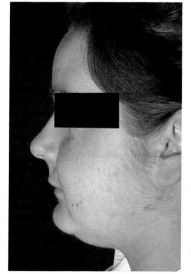

Fig. 63 Cushing's syndrome due to unilateral adenoma presenting with hirsutism and virilism.

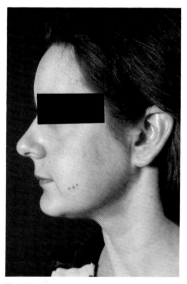

Fig. 64 Same patient 1 year following left adrenalectomy.

Diagnosis

24-hour urinary cortisol raised. Plasma cortisol at 9 a.m. after 2 mg of dexamethasone at midnight exceeds 250 nmol/l. Plasma ACTH raised or (inappropriately) normal in (1) and (3) (p. 37). Suppressed or undetectable in (2) and (4). Serum potassium low or normal in (1), (2), and (4) and almost invariably low in (3). X-ray of spine shows osteoporosis, especially in (1). Localisation of adenoma by CT scan or ultrasound, or by adrenal venous catheterisation and sampling. CT scan of the pituitary may identify adenoma.

Treatment

1. *Cushing's disease.* Ideally, selective transsphenoidal enucleation of microadenoma: less satisfactorily, either megavoltage pituitary irradiation or intrasellar yttrium implantation, with or without bilateral (total) adrenalectomy.
2. *Adrenal tumour.* Surgical removal (preferably retroperitoneal) after preoperative localisation. Adriamycin and adrenal blocking drugs (see below) of occasional value in inoperable adrenal carcinoma.
3. *Ectopic ACTH syndrome.* Rarely, excision of originating tumour is possible. Bilateral adrenalectomy or the use of adrenal-blocking drugs: metyrapone 1−2 g per day and/or aminoglutethimide 750−1500 mg per day.
4. *Iatrogenic Cushing's syndrome.* Corticosteroid side-effects minimised by alternate-day therapy and concurrent use of immunosuppressive drugs.

Complications

Untreated. Death from hypertensive complications and overwhelming infection. *Treated.* Adrenalectomy without surgery or radiotherapy to pituitary in (1) results in progressive pituitary enlargement in 30% of cases (*Nelson's syndrome*) resulting in pigmentation and progressive chiasmal compression, poorly responsive to all modes of therapy. Pituitary irradiation risks late development of hypopituitarism in approximately 10% of cases.

ADRENAL DISORDERS

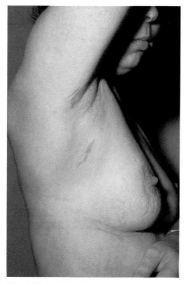

Fig. 65 Cushing's disease: active (pink) axillary striae.

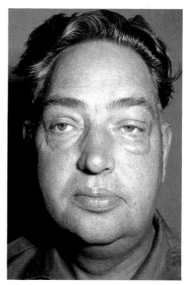

Fig. 66 Ectopic ATCH syndrome from medullary thyroid carcinoma: note conjunctival oedema.

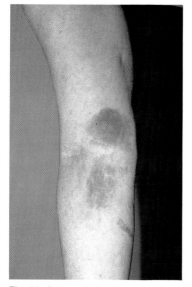

Fig. 67 Cushing's syndrome: thin skin and extensive bruising.

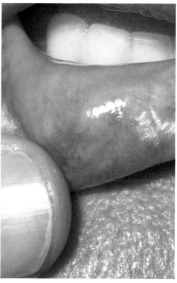

Fig. 68 Nelson's syndrome: pigmentation of lips (also seen in skin creases) 10 years after adrenalectomy for Cushing's disease.

Primary Adrenal Insufficiency
(Addison's Disease) (1)

Occurrence

Prevalence approximately 1 : 10 000.

Aetiology/ Pathogenesis

1. *Autoimmune destruction of adrenocortical cells.* Accounts for 90% of all cases of Addison's disease. Often in association with other familial disorders in the thyrogastric cluster (see pp. 3, 9, 15, 33, 93, 101). Linkage to HLA-B8, DR3 and DR4.
2. *Tuberculosis.* Previously common, now confined mainly to groups with high tuberculosis prevalence. Involvement of both adrenals usual, including adrenal medulla.
3. *Infiltrations.* Fungal infections, haemochromatosis, amyloidosis and metastatic carcinoma.
4. *Septicaemia.* With adrenal haemorrhage (Waterhouse-Friderichsen syndrome). Often associated with meningococcal septicaemia: usually fatal.
5. *Iatrogenic.* Bilateral adrenalectomy, or suppression of adrenal function by exogenous corticosteroids in the treatment of inflammatory disease.

Clinical features

In chronic cases (1, 2, 3), progressive anorexia, abdominal pain, weight loss and lethargy. Hypotension is common. Pigmentation in the buccal cavity, flexor skin creases, and points of solar exposure. Immune-associated vitiligo is often present. Other manifestations of underlying disorder apparent in (2) and (3). Acute adrenal insufficiency manifest by nausea, vomiting and dehydration, leading rapidly to shock, confusion and coma (Addisonian crisis), often precipitated by intercurrent stress (e.g. infection).

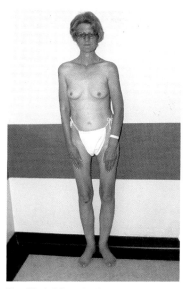

Fig. 69 Addison's disease: marked asthenia and pigmentation.

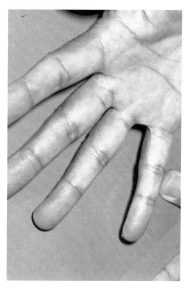

Fig. 70 Addison's disease: pigmentation of flexor skin creases.

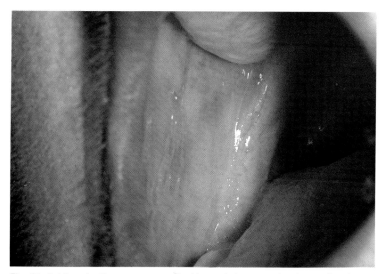

Fig. 71 Addison's disease: note typical buccal pigmentation immediately below finger: pigment was also present on lips and hands.

15 | Primary Adrenal Insufficiency
(Addison's Disease) (2)

Diagnosis

Screening test. Low plasma cortisol, failing to rise with tetracosactrin (Synacthen aqueous 250 μg i.m.) by more than 250 nmol/l.
Definitive test. 5-hour intravenous infusion of 500 μg tetracosactrin fails to stimulate cortisol and is diagnostic. Plasma ACTH invariably raised except with steroid therapy (5) where pituitary ACTH may also be suppressed. Adrenal antibodies in 80% of (1) and rare with (2), (3), (4). Abdominal X-ray shows adrenal calcification in 60% of tuberculous cases.

Treatment

Most cases require initial steroid 'loading'—hydrocortisone 100–300 mg daily orally or i.v., together with intravenous normal saline if dehydrated or shocked. Chronic replacement doses of hydrocortisone between 10 mg (children) and 30 mg (adults) daily, together with mineralocorticoid (fludrocortisone) 0.05–0.2 mg daily. Hydrocortisone dosage monitored by plasma cortisol day profile; fludrocortisone dosage ideally monitored by plasma renin estimation. With stress, all cases require tripling of hydrocortisone dosage, occasionally with parenteral administration.

Complications

Untreated. Progressive asthenia and death from shock.
Treated. Overdosage of hydrocortisone results in iatrogenic Cushing's syndrome (see p. 37). Overdosage of fludrocortisone produces fluid retention (oedema). Addisonian crisis occurs with failure to increase corticosteroid dose with stress in all aetiological groups.

ADRENAL DISORDERS

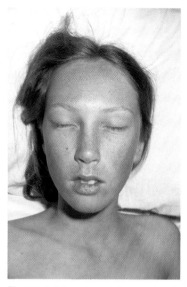

Fig. 72 Addisonian crisis: previously undiagnosed case precipitated by acute bronchitis.

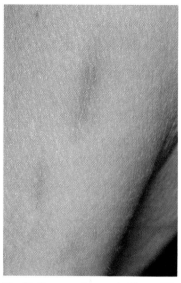

Fig. 73 Same patient as in Figure 72: pigmentation in area of scar.

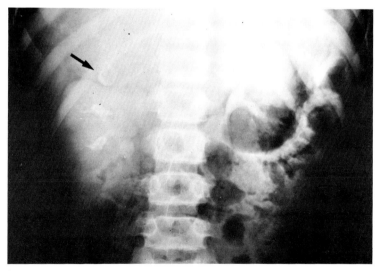

Fig. 74 Right adrenal calcification in 65-year-old patient with weight loss: adrenal carcinoma.

16 | Congenital Adrenal Hyperplasia

Occurence

Incidence approximately 1:8000 births.

**Aetiology/
Pathogenesis**

Congenital enzymatic defects in adrenal corticosteroid biosynthesis: deficient hydrocortisone synthesis results in ACTH hypersecretion with consequent adrenal hyperplasia. This results in partial (severe cases) or complete (mild cases) compensation for the defect, but with facilitation of additional metabolic pathways, particularly increasing androgen synthesis.

**Clinical
features**

21-hydroxylase defect. Commonest form: masculinisation, together with a salt-losing state (vomiting, dehydration) in the neonatal period in severe cases, or masculinisation alone later in life. Some male patients are undetected.
11-hydroxylase defect. Masculinisation and hypertension.
Other rare forms induce salt loss alone, lack of development of female sexual characteristics, or gross adrenal insufficiency incompatible with life.

Diagnosis

Elevated serum 17-hydroxyprogesterone and dehydro-epiandrosterone sulphate almost invariable. Plasma testosterone raised.

Treatment

In salt-losing cases, rehydration with saline and hydrocortisone administration. In older subjects, administration of hydrocortisone doses adequate to suppress abnormal steroidogenesis, together with use of mineralocorticoid (fludrocortisone) in some patients. Fully androgenised females presenting as physical and psychological males in adulthood are normally left untreated.

Complications

Untreated. Death from salt loss in infancy; physical and psychological sex reversal in childhood; infertility in all groups.
Treated. Iatrogenic Cushing's syndrome from overtreatment. Addisonian crisis due to inadequate steroid replacement with stress.

ADRENAL DISORDERS

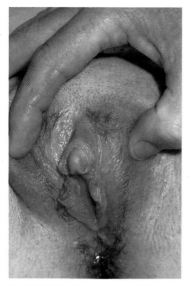

Fig. 75 Clitoral enlargement in a 13-year-old girl with CAH.

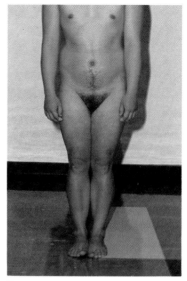

Fig. 76 17-year-old female with CAH: hirsutism and breast agenesis normalised following steroid replacement.

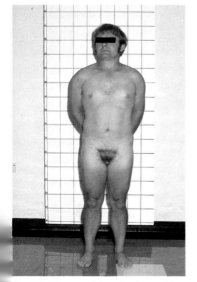

Fig. 77 32-year-old coal miner with infertility: 46 XX. Confirmed CAH not treated.

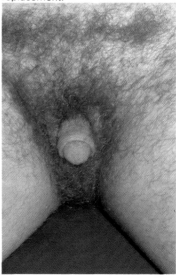

Fig. 78 Genital appearance of same patient as in Figure 77: enlarged phallus with hypospadias.

17 | Hyperaldosteronism
(Conn's Syndrome)

Occurrence

Prevalence less than 1 : 10 000 general population: between 0.1 and 0.5% of hypertensive population under age 50.

Aetiology/ Pathogenesis

In many cases, a benign unilateral adrenal aldosterone-producing adenoma: other cases have bilateral hyperplasia of adrenal zona glomerulosa. Occasionally familial.

Clinical features

Mild to moderate hypertension. Most cases are initially identified by the frequently, but not invariably associated hypokalaemia causing weakness and/or cardiac arrhythmias.

Diagnosis

Most adenoma patients have serum potassium less than 3.5 mmol/l, with mild metabolic alkalosis (serum bicarbonate > 28 mmol/l; blood pH 7.45–7.55). Plasma or urine aldosterone is raised, and non-suppressible by saline infusion or mineralocorticoid (fludrocortisone) loading. Plasma renin is low and not stimulated by erect posture or sodium depletion. Patients with hyperplasia have less marked abnormalities of biochemical parameters. Localisation of adenoma is by ultrasound, CT scan or retrograde femoral vein catheterisation and adrenal vein sampling.

Treatment

Adenoma. Unilateral partial or complete adrenalectomy. Medical treatment with spironolactone 100–400 mg daily is sometimes a satisfactory alternative.
Hyperplasia. Treatment with spironolactone as above.

Complications

Untreated. Hypokalaemia may induce tubular nephropathy and occasional death from arrhythmia.
Treated. Spironolactone induces gynaecomastia in males, polymenorrhoea in females.

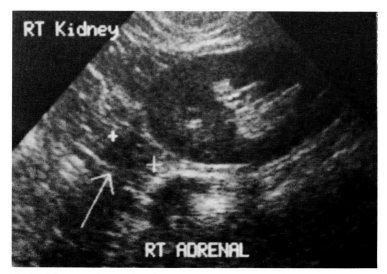

Fig. 79 Ultrasound scan showing 2.5 cm lesion in a 44-year-old woman with hypertension and hypokalaemia. Raised aldosterone, low renin.

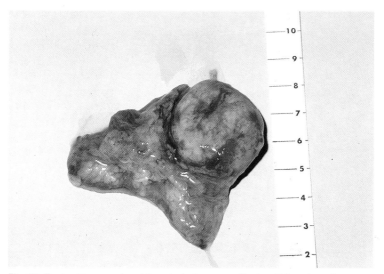

Fig. 80 Excised tumour (next to ruler) of same patient, within otherwise normal adrenal. Histology: aldosteronoma.

18 | Phaeochromocytoma

Occurrence

Prevalence below 1 : 10 000 of population: 0.1–0.5% of hypertensive patients under age 50.

Aetiology/ Pathogenesis

A usually benign tumour of chromaffin cells frequently arising from adrenal medulla and producing catecholamines (epinephrine, norepinephrine): less frequently (10%) in non-adrenal sites such as sympathetic ganglia, organ of Zuckerkandl or bladder. 10% of tumours are bilateral (especially common in children). Occasionally familial in association with medullary thyroid carcinoma (see p. 7), hyperparathyroidism and multiple mucosal neuromas (Sipple's syndrome or MEA type II or III; see p. 99).

Clinical features

Classically, paroxysmal hypertension associated with headache, palpitations, sweating, nausea, vomiting and occasionally collapse. Facial pallor and very high blood pressure during attacks. Episodes sometimes precipitated by physical exertion. Non-paroxysmal hypertension in up to 40% of cases, and postural hypotension often present. Sipple's patients have 'café au lait' skin spots and mucosal neuromas and/or findings of medullary thyroid carcinoma (see Fig. 12).

Diagnosis

Urinary vanillylmandelic acid (catecholamine metabolites) excretion is raised. More specifically, plasma catecholamines are elevated and non-suppressible by alpha-adrenergic agonists such as pentolinium or clonidine. Localisation of the tumour is achieved by CT scanning, and more specifically by isotope scanning after labelled metaiodobenzyl guanidine (MIBG-^{131}I).

Treatment

Surgical removal of tumour after localisation, plasma volume expansion, and usually alpha- and beta-adrenergic blocking drugs. Malignant cases are treated by catecholamine blocker metyrosine or high dose MIBG-[131]I.

Complications

Untreated. Most cases eventually fatal. *Treated.* Postoperative hypotension in inadequately prepared patients.

ADRENAL DISORDERS

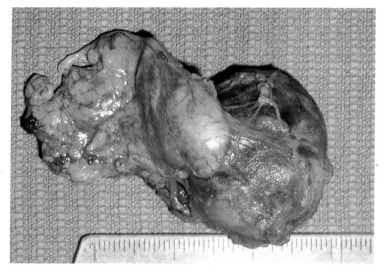

Fig. 81 5 cm vascular phaeochromocytoma; paler normal adrenal to the left. 50-year-old woman with collapse: blood pressure 240/160.

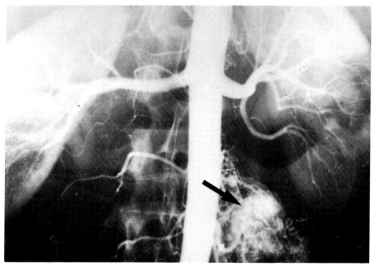

Fig. 82 Arteriogram of 40-year-old man with sustained hypertension (280/120). Angiography shows vascular phaeochromocytoma (arrow) arising from L2 sympathetic ganglion.

19 | Obesity

Occurrence	Prevalence 1 : 20 of most Western populations.
Aetiology/ Pathogenesis	Only rarely due to specific endocrinopathy (Cushing's syndrome, hypothyroidism, hypogonadism, hypothalamic disorders). Mostly a combination of excess calorie intake and decreased energy expenditure (exercise). Some individuals have abnormal external appetite cueing, or major psychiatric disturbance leading to overeating (bulimia). Increasing evidence for a genetic abnormality of thermogenesis in many cases.
Clinical features	Increase in body weight, dyspnoea, lethargy and secondary inactivity (see Complications, below).
Diagnosis	Definition arbitrary: life tables indicate significant risk when weight 20% above 'ideal'. Exclusion of endocrinopathies only indicated with specific clinical features (see pp. 1, 3, 25, 33, 37, 63)
Treatment	*Medical.* Increased physical activity, especially low-intensity, long-duration. Diet less than 1000 to 1500 calories, with high fibre, low fat content. Group therapy and behaviour modification sometimes of benefit. Anorexigenic drugs often habit forming and transient in effect. *Surgical.* In severe cases (50% above ideal weight), jaw wiring (dental fixation) coupled with a fluid diet allows excellent temporary weight loss, reversing in 90% of cases after unwiring. Gastric stapling or banding (to produce small gastric pouch/remnant) is effective therapy in gross obesity.
Complications	*Untreated.* Amenorrhoea, hypertension, ischaemic heart disease, osteoarthritis, diabetes mellitus, psychosocial disorders, pedestrian accidents. In gross cases, pulmonary hypoventilation with coma (Pickwickian syndrome). *Treated.* Habituation with drug therapy; gingival infection and caries with jaw wiring; selective food intolerance following gastric surgery.

METABOLIC DISORDERS

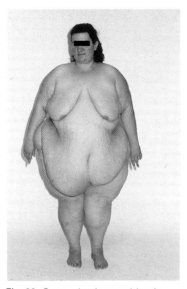

Fig. 83 Gross obesity resulting in Pickwickian syndrome.

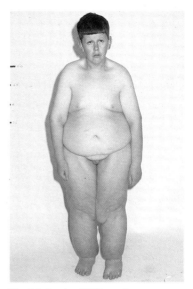

Fig. 84 Prader-Willi syndrome: obesity, hypogonadism, hypotonia and short stature.

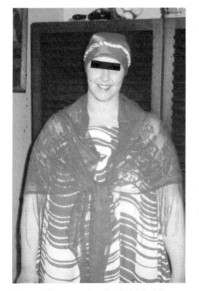

Fig. 85 Severe obesity (130 kg) in 28-year-old woman with hypertension (160/110).

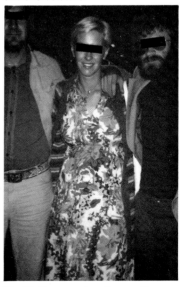

Fig. 86 Same patient 1 year after gastric bypass operation: weight 68 kg. Blood pressure 140/90.

20 Gonadal Dysgenesis
(Turner's Syndrome)

Occurrence

Incidence approximately 1:10 000 births.

Aetiology/Pathogenesis

Disorder determined by deficient short arm of second X-chromosome: most commonly a total absence of this chromosome due to meiotic non-disjunction (i.e. 45, X). Less frequently due to mosaicism (XO/XX or XO/XY) or other abnormality such as duplication (isochromosome) of the long arms of X.

Clinical features

In classical 45, X (Turner's) syndrome, amenorrhoea in phenotypic females with short stature, fibrous 'ovarian' streaks, webbed neck, shield chest, cubitus valgus, low hair line, ptosis, short 4th metacarpal and frequent association with aortic coarctation. Chromosome variants show less marked abnormality: functional gonadal tissue, absence of webbed neck and near normal stature. XY-cell line identifies a unilateral primitive gonad from which masculinisation is likely.

Diagnosis

Low serum oestradiol, elevated FSH and LH. Leucocyte karyotype reveals precise chromosomal complement; additional tissue karyotypes sometimes required to confirm mosaicism. Radiology reveals dysplastic bone and occasional true osteoporosis.

Treatment

Oestrogen replacement from age 14–18: additional cyclical progestogen minimises risk of uterine malignancy. Oxandrolone and synthetic growth hormone may accelerate long bone growth. Gonadectomy performed in XY mosaics in view of potential malignancy.

Complications

Untreated. Osteoporosis, increased risk of autoimmune thyroid disease.
Treated. Premature epiphyseal fusion with excess or early oestrogen replacement. Increased endometrial carcinoma with 'unopposed' oestrogen.

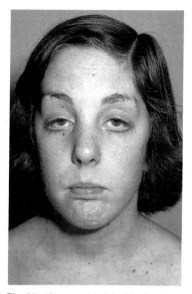

Fig. 87 18-year-old girl with classical (45, XO) gonadal dysgenesis: note ptosis, mild webbed neck and excess moles.

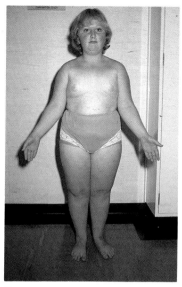

Fig. 88 18-year-old with XO/XX mosaic: cubitus valgus but no neck webbing.

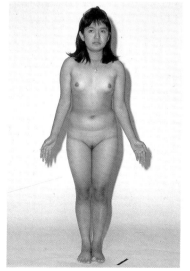

Fig. 89 17-year-old with isochromosome for long arm of X: minimal dwarfism.

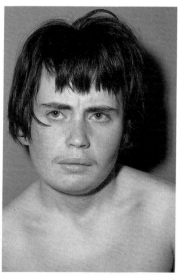

Fig. 90 15-year-old girl with gonadal dysgenesis mosaic (XO/XY): gonadoblastoma in unilateral ovotestis responsible for hirsutism.

21 | Testicular Feminisation Syndrome

Occurrence

Prevalence approximately 1 : 50 000.

Aetiology/ Pathogenesis

A familial disorder involving defective androgen binding to tissue receptors resulting in androgen resistance and consequent partial or complete feminisation.

Clinical features

Complete form. Total androgen resistance results in a phenotypic and psychosexual female; normal breasts and external genitalia, but reduced or absent axillary and pubic hair. Testes abdominal, inguinal or labial. Blind vagina.
Incomplete form. Partial androgen resistance results in phenotypic but occasionally psychosexually indeterminate females with ambiguous genitalia (partial labioscrotal fusion), clitoromegaly and mild hirsutism. Blind vagina.

Diagnosis

Karyotype normal male (46, XY). Serum testosterone normal: LH and FSH elevated due to defective feedback signal. Serum oestradiol high (for males). Principal differential diagnosis of 5-alpha-reductase deficiency.

Treatment

Complete. Gonadectomy performed after completion of puberty, followed by oestrogen therapy. Vaginal reconstruction rarely indicated.
Incomplete. Early gonadectomy and oestrogen replacement to avoid virilisation. Vaginal reconstruction often required.

Complications

Untreated. Malignant change in testes.
Treated. Psychological consequences of vaginal reconstruction.

FEMALE GONADAL DISORDERS

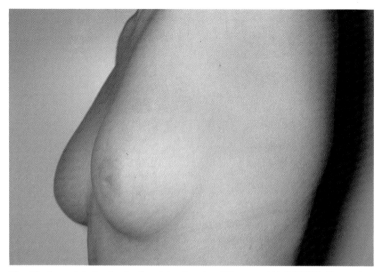

Fig. 91 Complete testicular feminisation in a 22-year-old 'girl' (XY). Normal breasts, no axillary hair.

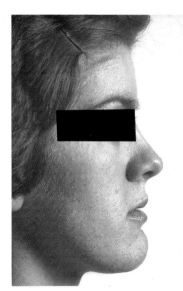

Fig. 92 Partial testicular feminisation (XY) in a 19-year-old hirsute 'girl'.

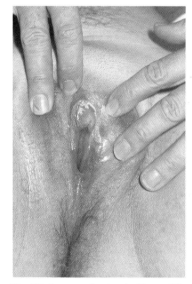

Fig. 93 Same patient as in Figure 92: clitoromegaly and partial (posterior) labioscrotal fusion.

Hirsutism (Benign Androgen Excess/Stein-Leventhal Syndrome) (1)

Occurrence

Prevalence approximately 1 : 80 females.

Aetiology/ Pathogenesis

Increased androgen production largely from the ovary; altered steroid biosynthesis arising from abnormally stimulated thecal cells in non-maturing follicles, which undergo cystic change. Primary defect unknown, but may be of hypothalamic or gonadal origin. Suggestive association with maternal androgen administration in some patients. Often familial.

Clinical features

Wide spectrum. Most cases have history of hirsutism extending from puberty, affecting upper lip, chin, sideburns, breasts, abdominal wall and thighs, with or without acne, greasy hair and skin. Occasional patients have acne only. Menstrual pattern occasionally normal with confirmed regular ovulation; oligomenorrhoea and complete amenorrhoea in some patients. When associated with obesity, infertility and demonstrably polycystic ovaries, identified as Stein-Leventhal syndrome.

Diagnosis

Serum testosterone normal or elevated; SHBG reduced. Accordingly free (measured or derived) testosterone levels invariably elevated. LH high, FSH low and serum oestradiol normal. Serum progesterone levels usually follicular-phase confirming anovulation despite regular menstruation. Laparoscopy or ultrasound confirms polycystic ovaries in some severe cases.

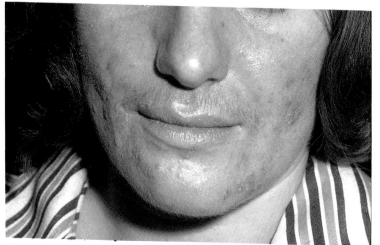

Fig. 94 Benign androgen excess: note acne, hirsutism and seborrhoea. Ovaries normal on ultrasound.

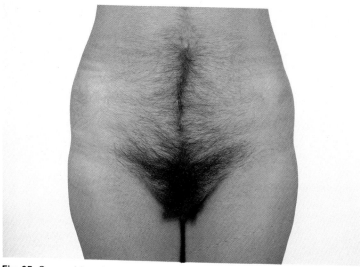

Fig. 95 Severe hirsutism in benign androgen excess: hair also present on low back, upper lip, chin and breasts.

Differential diagnosis

Other androgenic lesions almost invariably associated with amenorrhoea and true virilism (breast atrophy, muscular hypertrophy, deep voice, clitoromegaly):

a. *Congenital adrenal hyperplasia.* Late presenting; 17-hydroxyprogesterone and DHAS confirm.
b. *Hilus cell tumours.* Benign lesions of ovary, with similar findings to benign androgen excess. Laparotomy or laparoscopy required for diagnosis.
c. *Arrhenoblastoma.* Rare masculinising tumour of ovary: some cases associated with hypertension. Ultrasound may be diagnostic.
d. *Virilising tumours of adrenal.* Adenoma/carcinoma.

Treatment

Hirsutism. Mild cases treated with electrolysis, depilatory creams, waxes and bleaches. Exogenous oestrogen suppresses androgen production by LH and FSH suppression, and reduces receptor sensitivity. Usually given as contraceptive pill using low-androgenic progestogen (e.g. desogestrel). Low dose corticosteroids are occasionally of value. Severe cases treated with anti-androgens; spironolactone 100–200 mg daily or cyproterone acetate 150 mg daily in reverse cycle with ethinyloestradiol.
Infertility. Clomiphene citrate 25–50 mg on day 5–9 induces LH surge and ovulation in many non-ovulating patients. Pulsatile GnRH infusion or ovarian wedge resection sometimes required.

Complications

Untreated. Increasing hirsutism, rupture of follicular cysts, infertility.
Treated. Corticosteroid and oestrogen side-effects. Spironolactone induces transient diuresis and polymenorrhoea. Cyproterone occasionally produces tiredness. Clomiphene may induce nausea together with multiple ovulation when used in large doses.

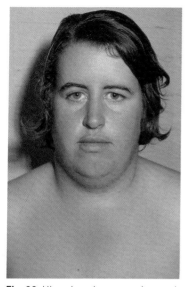

Fig. 96 Hirsutism, hypertension and amenorrhoea. Testosterone elevated. Arrhenoblastoma removed at laparotomy.

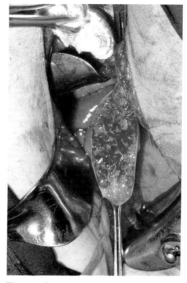

Fig. 97 Stein-Leventhal syndrome. Polycystic ovaries at laparotomy. Patient was hirsute, obese and amenorrhoeic.

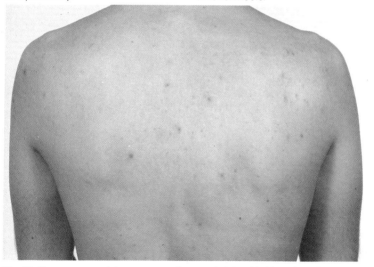

Fig. 98 Severe acne, also present on face and chest. No hirsutism. Free testosterone elevated. Complete resolution obtained with spironolactone.

23 | **Anorexia Nervosa** (Chronic Hypothalamic Anovulation)

Occurrence

Prevalence 1 : 100−1000. Female : male ratio 20 : 1.

Aetiology/ Pathogenesis

Hypogonadotrophic hypogonadism secondary to psychological disturbance with stress-induced inhibition of hypothalmaic GnRH release. Weight reduction (usually to below 40 kg) further inhibits GnRH release due to unknown mechanisms.

Clinical features

Mildest cases have only stress-induced anovulation with or without amenorrhoea. History of alternating binge-eating and fasting in some cases with or without striking weight changes. True anorexia nervosa manifest by reduced food intake, self-induced vomiting and purgation, together with physical hyperactivity, often quite elusive, without obvious gross psychiatric disturbance. Weight reduction below 40 kg almost always present.

Diagnosis

Low serum FSH, LH and oestradiol (testosterone in males). Fasting serum growth hormone and cortisol elevated.

Treatment

Counselling and support with reassurance in mild cases. Psychiatric therapy in true anorexia nervosa: no indication for endocrine therapy.

Complications

Untreated. Overt depression supervenes in some cases with suicidal tendency. Osteoporosis and increased susceptibility to infection in older patients.
Treated. Nil.

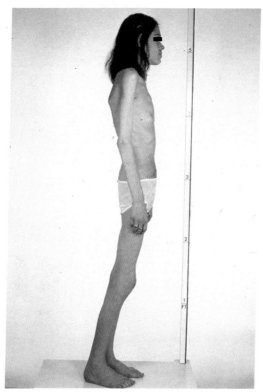

Fig. 99 Anorexia nervosa in a 22-year-old girl. No axillary or pubic hair was present.

24 | Kallman's Syndrome (Organic Hypogonadotrophic Hypogonadism)

Occurrence

Prevalence below 1 : 50 000. Male : female ratio 6 : 1.

Aetiology/ Pathogenesis

An abnormality in hypothalamic function resulting in deficient GnRH stimulation of LH and FSH release, coupled to olfactory, auditory or optic nerve defects. No structural abnormalities have been identified.

Clinical features

Hypogonadism (and infertility) with normal longitudinal growth. Usually presenting as delayed (absent) puberty. Anosmia (or hyposmia) often only on direct questioning. Colour blindness and mild nerve deafness occasionally associated. Gynaecomastia rare. Testes small and soft in males; breasts underdeveloped in females.

Diagnosis

Karyotype normal (XY or XX); serum FSH, LH and testosterone (oestradiol) low. Gonadotrophin level occasionally unresponsive to GnRH infusion, but recruited response demonstrable with repeated stimulation.

Treatment

Gonadal hormone replacement as appropriate (testosterone oenanthate 250 mg i.m. every 2−4 weeks or ethinyl-oestradiol 30 mg daily with norethisterone 5 mg for 5 days to produce withdrawal bleeding). Fertility often induceable with pulsatile GnRH, or less satisfactorily with gonadotrophin therapy.

Complications

Untreated. Osteoporosis.
Treated. Multiple ovulation with use of gonadotrophins in infertility management.

MALE GONADAL DISORDERS

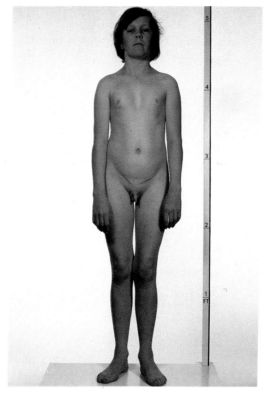

Fig. 100 Kallman's syndrome in a 24-year-old man. Eunuchoid proportions, absent body hair and small testes. Complete anosmia.

25 | Klinefelter's Syndrome

Occurrence

Incidence 1:1000 male births.

Aetiology/ Pathogenesis

A chromosomal disorder arising from meiotic non-dysjunction and commonly resulting in a 47, XXY karyotype. Testicular Leydig-cell hyperplasia and hyalinisation of seminiferous tubules are disease hallmarks.

Clinical features

Absence or delayed development of male secondary sex characteristics; small firm testes, mostly associated with gynaecomastia. Infertility and impotence almost invariable. Eunuchoid proportions (span exceeds height; sole-pubis exceeds crown-pubis). Mosaics (XXY/XY: XXY/XYY most commonly) have less striking clinical features and may have limited fertility. Increased association with mental subnormality, diabetes and autoimmune thyroid disease.

Diagnosis

Buccal smear shows Barr bodies (supernumerary X-chromosome). Leucocyte karyotype reveals chromosomal complement. Serum testosterone low; LH and FSH elevated Major differential diagnosis is *Reifenstein's syndrome*—gynaecomastia, hypospadias, normal (XY) karyotype—a syndrome probably due to partial tissue androgen resistance.

Treatment

Androgen replacement, most commonly testosterone oenanthate 250 mg every 2−4 weeks stimulates sexual development and potency: fertility unaffected. Mammectomy often cosmetically indicated.

Complications

Untreated. Earlier onset osteoporosis, increased risk of breast carcinoma.
Treated. Nil.

MALE GONADAL DISORDERS

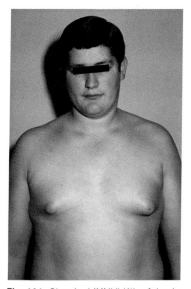

Fig. 101 Classical (XXY) Klinefelter's syndrome. Absent beard growth and frontal hair recession.

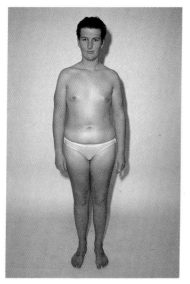

Fig. 102 Klinefelter's mosaic (XXY/XY). Small genitalia, minimal gynaecomastia. Presented with infertility.

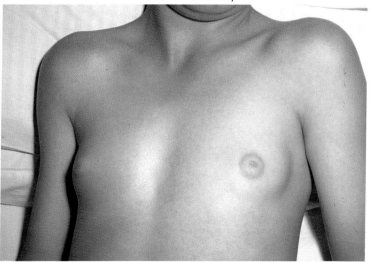

Fig. 103 13-year-old presenting with gynaecomastia and history of violent behaviour. XXY/XYY Klinefelter's mosaic confirmed.

26 | Gynaecomastia

Occurrence
Incidence 1 : 50 males at some time in life.

Aetiology/ Pathogenesis
True duct epithelial hypertrophy of one or both breasts, associated with specific entities:
Neo-natal. Due to transplacental oestrogen passage.
Pubertal. Oestrogen 'surge' consequent on aromatisation of increasing androgen concentration.
Senile. Increased oestrogen/androgen ratio postulated.
Drugs. Oestrogens, digoxin, spironolactone, methyl-dopa, phenothiazines.
Endocrinopathies. Klinefelter's and Reifenstein's syndrome: hyperthyroidism.
Tumours. Ectopic gonadotrophin production (commonly oat-cell carcinoma): chorio- and Leydig-cell carcinoma.
Diverse. Hepatic cirrhosis, renal failure, re-feeding after under-nutrition.

Clinical features
Disc-like or diffuse breast enlargement of one or both breasts, rarely painful unless acutely developing. In neonatal and pubertal cases invariably self-limiting; drug-induced cases mostly reversible, other clinical features relating to underlying disease.

Diagnosis
Investigations usually unhelpful; history and examination usually provided diagnosis.

Treatment
Removal of underlying cause. Expectant policy in neonatal and pubertal cases. Clomiphene or danazol occasionally effective in persisting pubertal gynaecomastia. Mammectomy indicated when painful or unsightly.

Complications
Untreated. Embarrassment and self-consciousness.
Treated. None.

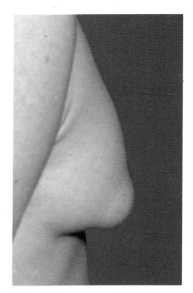

Fig. 104 Gynaecomastia due to spironolactone therapy. Complete regression after discontinuing drug.

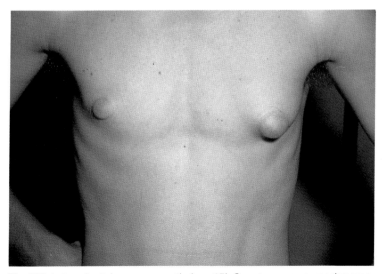

Fig. 105 Late pubertal gynaecomastia (age 15). Spontaneous regression was seen by age 18.

27 | **Precocious Puberty**

Occurrence
Onset of puberty before age 8 in 1 : 5000.

Aetiology/ Pathogenesis
True sexual precocity. Sexual and reproductive maturity secondary to hypothalamic dysfunction: rarely due to primary hypothyroidism. In 20% of males, underlying tumour (pinealoma, hamartoma, glioma, craniopharyngioma); in females less common.
Albright's syndrome. Precocious puberty associated with polyostotic fibrous dysplasia of bone and patchy brown skin pigmentation.
Precocious pseudo-puberty. A primary pathological adrenal or gonadal excess of androgen or oestrogen.
a. *Male congentital adrenal hyperplasia* (CAH)
b. *Tumours.* Teratoma or seminoma of testis in males; teratoma or thecal-cell ovarian tumour in females.

Clinical features
Initial rapid growth, later short stature due to epiphyseal fusion. In true precocity, menstruation (and fertility) closely follows breast and genital hair development. In pseudo-puberty, often infertile.

Diagnosis
Serum oestradiol or testosterone high. Gonadotrophins high with teratoma, normal in true precocity and suppressed in pseudo-puberty. 17-hydroxyprogesterone elevated in CAH. X-rays reveal bone cysts in Albright's syndrome. Advanced bone age in most cases. CT scan identifies hypothalamic tumours: EEG often abnormal in true sexual precocity.

Treatment
That of underlying abnormality. Cyproterone acetate and medroxyprogesterone occasionally effective. High dose GnRH suppresses gonadotrophin release.

Complications
Untreated. Self-consciousness, embarrassment and complications of the underlying disease.
Treated. Complications of neurosurgery or irradiation.

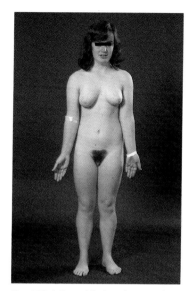

Fig. 106 Idiopathic (true) precocious puberty (age 9): mother's age at puberty was 11.

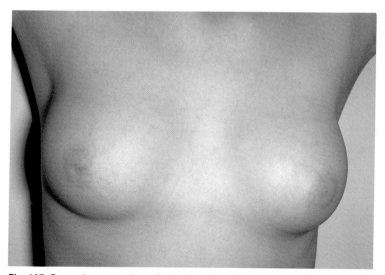

Fig. 107 Precocious pseudo-puberty: breast enlargement age 10; no sexual hair present; small ovarian theca-cell tumour.

28 | Simple Delayed Puberty
(Small Delay Syndrome)

Occurrence

Incidence approximately 1 : 500. Male : Female ratio 6 : 1.

Aetiology/ Pathogenesis

Defined as onset of puberty beyond age 15. Unknown aetiology. Often familial, inherited from isosexual parent. No demonstrable anatomical lesion. Mechanism of associated delay in longitudinal growth unknown.

Clinical features

Fall off in growth velocity often before age 10 and usually more prominent in boys. Testes small in males, breasts undeveloped in females; lack of sexual hair in both sexes. Embarrassment and self-consciousness common.

Diagnosis

Growth velocity < 5 cm per annum usual. Bone age (Greulich-Pyle: Tanner-Whitehouse methods) usually delayed 2 years or more behind chronological age. Serum testosterone, LH and FSH all low. Differential diagnosis: exclusion of other causes of short stature (see p. 73) and hypogonadotrophic hypogonadism (see p. 63).

Treatment

Uncommonly requires treatment: catch-up growth is invariable and ultimate mature height normal. If socially indicated, puberty is induceable by intramuscular chorionic gonadotrophin 1500 units twice weekly for 6 weeks, or alternatively testosterone or GnRH therapy.

Complications

Untreated. Nil.
Treated. Premature epiphyseal fusion if treated with excessive androgen or gonadotrophin dosage.

PUBERTY AND GROWTH DISORDERS

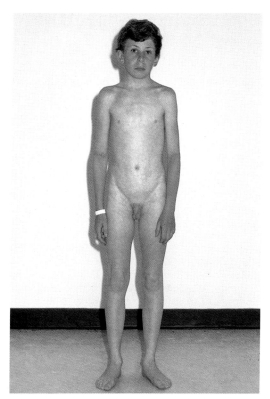

Fig. 108 Delayed puberty (small delay syndrome) (age 18). Note short stature, lack of pubic hair and muscle development. Father's puberty also delayed.

Occurrence

Usually of social/medical significance when child is below 3rd percentile for age, i.e. incidence 3 in 100 of population under age 18 (see Appendix 2, pp. 105–106).

Aetiology/ Pathogenesis

Growth hormone deficiency. Idiopathic (presumptive hypothalamic disorder) in the majority of cases; secondary to craniopharyngioma or other structural abnormality (i.e. septo-optic dysplasia) in the remainder.

Laron dwarfism. Growth hormone resistance due to somatomedin receptor defect.

Hypothyroidism (see p. 1). Usually autoimmune thyroiditis.

Cushing's syndrome (see p. 37). Suppression of bone growth due to inhibition of somatomedin action and suppression of pituitary growth hormone release.

Small delay syndrome (delayed puberty) (see p. 71). Delayed maturation of hypothalamic releasing centres.

Psychosocial deprivation. Extreme emotional and social upheaval resulting in 'functional' suppression of hypothalamic growth hormone releasing factors.

Anorexia nervosa (see p. 61). Due to hypothalamic 'turn-off'.

Gonadal dysgenesis (Turner's syndrome) (see p. 53). Short stature due to dysplastic bone, hyporesponsive to growth factors.

Precocious puberty (see p. 69). Initial growth rate stimulus, later short stature due to premature epiphyseal fusion.

Prader-Willi syndrome. congenital hypothalamic lesion with associated abnormalities (see Fig. 84).

Laurence-Moon-Biedl syndrome. Congenital hypothalamic syndrome with retinitis pigmentosa and polydactyly.

Pseudohypoparathyroidism. Renal tubular resistance to parathormone action.

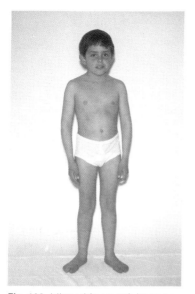

Fig. 109 Idiopathic growth hormone deficiency (age 11): symmetric short stature. Responded to hGH therapy.

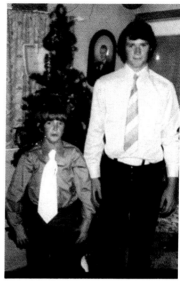

Fig. 110 Twins (non-identical) aged 17. Boy on left had idiopathic growth hormone deficiency.

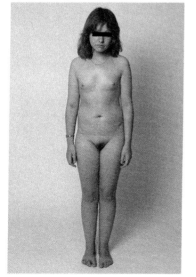

Fig. 111 Short stature due to anorexia nervosa (age 18). In remission at time of photograph.

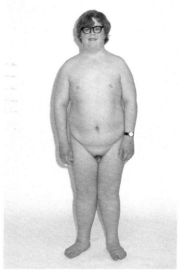

Fig. 112 Atypical Laurence-Moon-Biedl syndrome: short stature, retinitis pigmentosa but no polydactyly.

Aetiology/
Pathogenesis
(cont)

Other short stature syndromes not associated
with demonstrable endocrine abnormality:
Familial short stature. Inherited genetic factors.
Small-for-dates (intrauterine growth retardation).
Mechanism uncertain, possibly involving
placental insufficiency, without catch-up growth.
Chronic illness. Congenital cardiac disease,
chronic obstructive or infective pulmonary
disease (interfering with oxygenation), chronic
renal failure.
Malabsorption syndrome. Commonly coeliac
disease (gluten-sensitive enteropathy) or
giardiasis.
Rare named syndromes of bone development.
Russell-Silver *dwarfism:* cause unknown.
Achondroplasia and other dyschondroplastic
syndromes.

Clinical
features

Highly diverse. Careful history identifies
precocious puberty, parental pubertal delay,
psychological and social factors as well as
anorexia nervosa. Birth weight identifies
intrauterine growth redardation. Symmetrical
(proportional) dwarfism suggests systemic
illness, malabsorption, familial short stature,
growth hormone deficiency, small delay and
intrauterine growth retardation.

Special clinical features identify
Hypothyroidism. Coarse features, short limbs,
sallow complexion.
Prader-Willi syndrome. Hypotonia, obesity,
hypogonadism.
Laurence-Moon-Biedl syndrome. Retinitis
pigmentosa, polydactyly.
Septo-optic dysplasia. Optic atrophy and other
neurological abnormalities.
Gonadal dysgenesis. Neck webbing, cubitus
valgus.

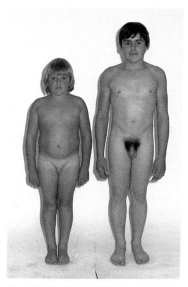

Fig. 113 Brothers with spondyloepiphyseal dysplasia: note short trunk but normal length limbs.

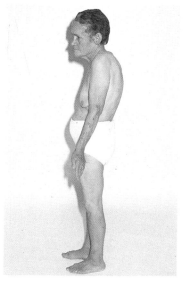

Fig. 114 Pseudohypoparathyroidism: note marked kyphosis; marked mental retardation present.

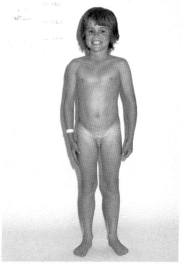

Fig. 115 12-year-old with gluten-sensitive enteropathy: height 8 cm below 3rd percentile. Note absence of emaciation: prompt growth response to gluten-free diet.

Clinical
features
(cont)

Systemic illness. Cardiac, pulmonary, renal abnormalities.
Cushing's syndrome. Obesity, striae, hypertension.
Russell-Silver dwarfism. Limb asymmetry, pixieface.
Achondroplasia. Short limbs and spine.
Spondyloepiphyseal dysplasia. Short spine, long limbs.
Pseudohypoparathyroidism. Brachydactyly, mental retardation.
Anorexia nervosa. See p. 61.
Precocious puberty. See p. 69.

Diagnosis

Skeletal X-rays identify bony abnormalities: usually confirms bone age delayed in most cases except precocious puberty. Evidence of intracranial calcification (pseudohypoparathyroidism and craniopharyngioma). Exercising (stress) hGH (normal > 20 mU/l) is screening test for hGH deficiency: definitive testing with insulin-induced hypoglycaemia. Serum T4, T3 and 24-hour urinary cortisol as appropriate.

Treatment

Growth hormone deficiency treated with natural or synthetic human growth hormone: some cases of gonadal dysgenesis, small delay and constitutional short stature may also respond. Small delay syndrome may be treated with chorionic gonadotrophin or androgens (see p. 71). Cushing's syndrome and hypothyroidism (see pp. 37 and 1 respectively): effective treatment of underlying illness should restore growth velocity.

Complications

Untreated. Those of the underlying condition.
Treated. No complications if appropriate therapy used.

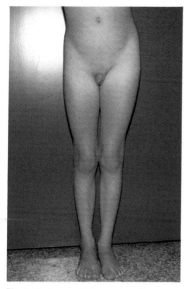

Fig. 116 Russell-Silver dwarfism: note asymmetric limb length.

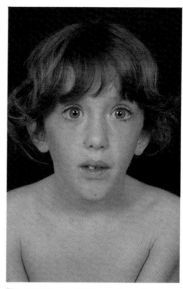

Fig. 117 Russell-Silver dwarfism: characteristic facial (pixie) appearance.

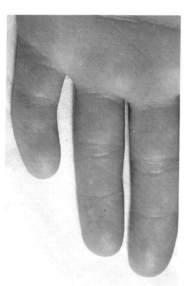

Fig. 118 Clinodactyly, a key feature of Russell-Silver dwarfism: may be a normal finding.

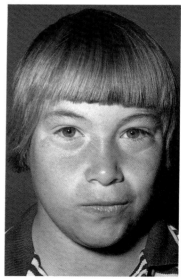

Fig. 119 Juvenile hypothyroidism presenting with short stature: sallow pigmentation due to carotenaemia.

Primary Hyperparathyroidism (1)

Occurrence

Prevalence approximately 1 : 1000 over age 20.

Aetiology/ Pathogenesis

In 80% of cases, a single parathyroid adenoma, occasionally familial and in association with other tumours (pituitary, pancreatic in Werner's syndrome, MEA type I; phaeochromocytoma and C-cell carcinoma in MEA type II or III; see p. 99), causes unknown. In 15% of cases, multiple gland hyperplasia. In 5% of cases, carcinoma of parathyroid.

Clinical features

Most mild cases asymptomatic, identified on routine biochemical screening. Higher serum calcium (above 3.0 mmol/1) may be associated with dyspepsia, bone pain (demineralisation), pathological fractures, arthropathies (including pseudogout), general malaise, myopathy and ultimately renal failure (nephrocalcinosis). Ectopic calcium deposition on cornea, conjunctivae and tympanic membrane, clinically detectable in some cases.

Diagnosis

Serum calcium elevated, serum phosphate reduced. Serum alkaline phosphatase elevated if significant bone involvement present. Serum parathormone elevated (C-terminal assay) or inappropriately detectable in most cases (other hypercalcaemia causes suppressed parathormone). Hyperchloraemic acidosis (serum chloride > 107, bicarbonate < 24 mmo/l) often present. Renal function studies show decreased tubular function (concentration defect) and later decreased glomerular function. Bone X-rays show generalised demineralisation or cystic changes (osteitis fibrosa cystica). Slit lamp examination displays ectopic corneal calcification. Adenoma localised by preoperative double isotope scanning or by venography with sampling to identify pathological hormone gradient.

METABOLIC BONE DISEASE

don't confuse ē myeloma!

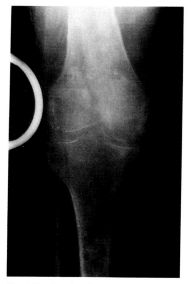 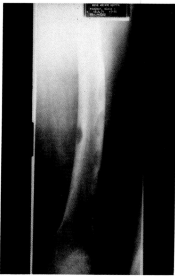

Fig. 120 Osteitis fibrosa cystica presenting as painful knee: cystic change and resorption in tibia and fibula.

Fig. 121 60-year-old patient with nausea: serum calcium 3.5 mmol/1. Asymptomatic osteitis fibrosa cystica in femur.

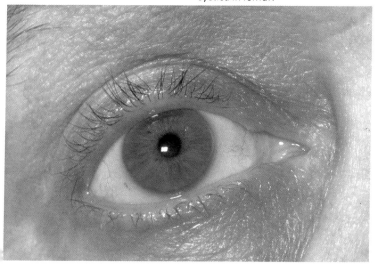

Fig. 122 Band keratopathy (corneal calcification) in hyperparathyroidism: crescentic white deposit on medial limbus of cornea.

Differential diagnosis

Sarcoidosis. Serum calcium, phosphate elevated: other evidence of sarcoidosis identifiable.
Multiple myelomatosis. Bone tenderness, abnormal protein electrophoresis.
Ectopic PTH syndrome. Hypokalaemic alkalosis associated (serum potassium < 3.5, chloride < 98, bicarbonate > 28 mmol/l). Serum PTH suppressed.
Vitamin D overdosage. Calcium and phosphate elevated, and history confirmatory.
Multiple bone metastases. Bone scan identifies multiple hot spots.
Hypothyroidism, hyperthyroidism, acromegaly, Addison's disease. All may induce hypercalcaemia (see individual disorders).
Milk-alkali syndrome. History confirms.

Treatment

Operative. Excision of adenoma by skilled surgeon. Hyperplasia managed by excision of all enlarged glands and either partial removal of remaining glands, or by reimplantation of excised tissue in forearm.
Non-operative. Asymptomatic cases may justify observation only. Rehydration, oral and/or intravenous sodium phosphate or sulphate together with frusemide used for temporary control. Carcinoma unresponsive to radiotherapy and most cytotoxic agents.

Complications

Untreated. Progressive but variable deterioration of tubular and glomerular function with irreversible renal failure. Progressive and variable loss of bone mass with related symptoms.
Treated. Unsuccessful location of adenoma: hypoparathyroidism postoperatively—either temporary due to 'hungry' bones, or permanent due to accidental damage to remaining parathyroid tissue.

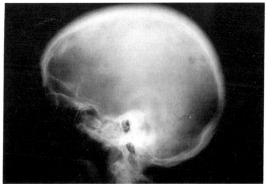

Fig. 123 Cystic lesion in skull due to multiple myeloma (serum calcium 4.1 mmol/l). Differential diagnosis includes primary hyperparathyroidism.

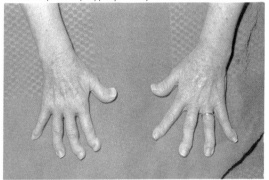

Fig. 124 Extensive terminal phalangeal destruction and deformity due to primary hyperparathyroidism.

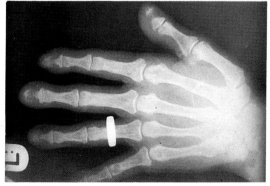

Fig. 125 X-ray of same patient: note multiple terminal phalangeal 'pseudo' fractures due to bone resorption.

Occurrence

Nutritional cause in up to 1 : 10 in some populations. Other forms uncommon.

Aetiology/ Pathogenesis

Deficiency, abnormal metabolism or defective target organ action of vitamin D or phosphate.

a. *Nutritional vitamin D deficit*. Especially common in developing countries, and in the elderly.
b. *Defective solar exposure*. Common in black ethnic groups emigrating to cloudier climates.
c. *Malabsorption syndrome/steatorrhea*. Glutensensitive enteropathy, regional ileitis, gastrointestinal surgery, biliary cirrhosis.
d. *Chronic liver disease*. Defective 25-hydroxylation of vitamin D.
e. *Anticonvulsant therapy*. Abnormal hydroxylation of vitamin D.
f. *Pseudo vitamin D resistant rickets*. Defective renal dihydroxylation of 25-hydroxy vitamin D
g. *Chronic renal failure*. Defective 1, 25-hydroxylation of vitamin D together with phosphate retention resulting in secondary hyperparathyroidism and renal osteodystrophy.
h. *Chronic purgative abuse*. Phosphate depletion.
i. *Aluminium hydroxide ingestion*. Phosphate depletion.
j. *Renal tubular acidosis*. Abnormal renal phosphate loss.
k. *Fanconi syndrome*. Abnormal renal phosphate loss.
l. *Vitamin D-resistant rickets*. Familial renal phosphate transport defect.
m. *Diphosphonate and fluoride therapy*. Inhibit 1, 25-dihydroxy-vitamin D action on bone.

Clinical features

In *infancy and childhood* (rickets), growth retardation, neuromuscular irritability (due to hypocalcaemia), skeletal thinning and deformity. In *adults* (osteomalacia), symptoms occasionally lacking, or clinical picture dominated by underlying disease. Severe cases have back pain, bone deformity and pathological fractures.

METABOLIC BONE DISEASE

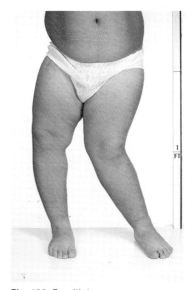

Fig. 126 Familial hypophosphataemic rickets: 'windswept' valgum/varum deformity. Patient was also short.

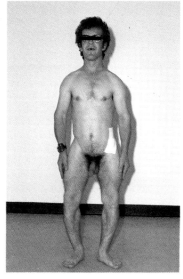

Fig. 127 Vitamin D-resistant rickets. Note leg shortening.

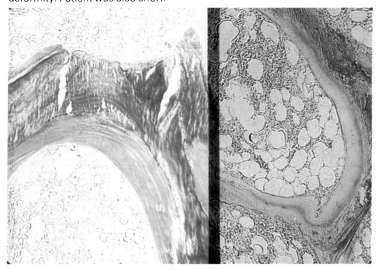

Fig. 128 Bone biopsies showing (left) laminated thickened, uncalcified osteoid seams (light blue) of osteomalacia. Repeat biopsy (right) shows narrowed osteoid seams 6 months after vitamin D.

31 | Rickets and Osteomalacia (2)

Diagnosis

Typical cases have hypocalcaemia and hypophosphataemia with elevated serum alkaline phosphatase (secondary hyperparathyroidism). Serum 25-hydroxy-vitamin D levels low in a, b, c, d, e. Serum 1, 25-dihydroxy-vitamin D low in f, g (and also usually in a, b, c, d, e). Marked hypophosphataemia usually with normal serum vitamin D metabolite levels in h, i, j, k, l. Fanconi syndrome patients have glycosuria, aminoaciduria and proteinuria and may be secondary to other causes such as lead intoxication. Radiology in children shows cuffed epiphyses and flared distal long bones, non-closure of calvarial sutures and defective dentition. In adults, reduced bone density with pseudo-fractures (symmetrical zones of decalcification in scapulae, femora and pubic-ischial rami). Bone biopsy shows widened unmineralised osteoid seams irrespective of aetiology.

Prevention

Maintenance of sunlight exposure in elderly, especially immigrant blacks. Adequate oral intake of vitamin D: supplements may be indicated.

Treatment

Calcitriol (1, 25-hydroxy-vitamin D) 0.25−0.5 µg daily plus calcium supplements. Vitamin D resistance and hypophosphataemic rickets require 10−20 times the above dosages with or without supplemental phosphate: corrective orthopaedic surgery frequently required. Parathyroidectomy for autonomous adenoma development in renal osteodystrophy.

Complications

Untreated. Progressive bone deformity and pain. *Treated.* Hypercalcaemia and renal failure secondary to vitamin D overdosage.

METABOLIC BONE DISEASE

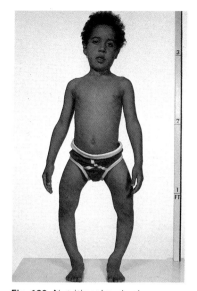

Fig. 129 Nutritional and solar vitamin D-deficiency rickets in a 9-year-old.

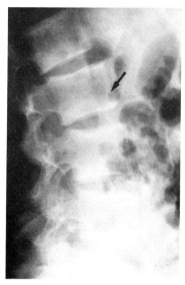

Fig. 130 'Rugger jersey' spine of renal osteodystrophy. Note osteosclerosis (arrow).

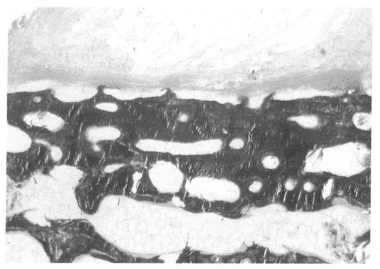

Fig. 131 Iliac crest biopsy in secondary hyperparathyroidism (renal osteodystrophy). Note scalloping and tunnelling due to osteoclastic resorption.

32 | Paget's Disease of Bone
(Osteitis Deformans)

Occurrence

Radiological involvement 1 : 10—20 over age 60.

Aetiology/ Pathogenesis

Occasionally familial monostotic or polyostotic involvement of skeleton. Increased vascularity and osteoclastic rarefaction is followed by deformity and subsequent osteoblastic sclerosis, with persistence of arteriovenous intraosseous shunts. Viral or autoimmune aetiology is possible in some cases.

Clinical features

Most cases are asymptomatic. Deformity and bowing of long bones, especially tibia, femora with joint pain in juxta-articular disease. Classical appearance of skull with frontal bossing, headache and hearing loss due to auditory nerve compression. Other nerve compression syndromes seen especially in spinal Paget's disease. Polyostotic disease sometimes associated with gross arteriovenous shunting and hyperdynamic circulation leading to cardiac failure.

Diagnosis

Clinical features may be diagnostic. Alkaline phosphatase grossly elevated in polyostotic disease. Isotope bone scan is the most sensitive technique for documenting extent of multiple bone disease. Radiology identifies abnormal lesions. Serum calcium mostly normal, but elevated when immobilisation of polyostotic Paget's disease patients occurs.

Treatment

Calcitonin (salmon or human synthetic) suppresses osteoblastic activity and reduces bone pain. The cytotoxic drug mithromycin acts similarly. Diphosphonates reduce bone turnover.

Complications

Untreated. Fibrosarcomatous change in 5—10% of cases. Progressive pain and disability and cardiac failure.
Treated. Mithromycin induces bone marrow suppression: diphosphonate may produce osteomalacia.

METABOLIC BONE DISEASE

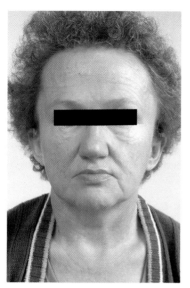

Fig. 132 Paget's disease of skull: typical frontal bone bossing. Patient complained of severe constant headache.

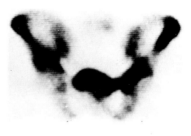

Fig. 133 Bone scan of extensive Paget's disease of pelvis: involved areas show black.

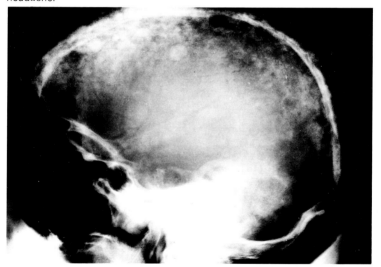

Fig. 134 Lateral skull X-ray in Paget's disease: mottled expansion of calvarium.

Osteoporosis (1)

Occurrence

Prevalence approximately 1:30 over age 60.

Aetiology/ Pathogenesis

Overall loss of bone mass, including osteoid matrix, resulting in bone pain and pathological fracture. Age-related decline in bone mass recordable in all populations.
Cushing's syndrome. Due to hypercatabolism.
Hyperthyroidism. Due to hypercatabolism.
Male hypogonadism. Due to decreased bone formation.
Post-menopausal. Due to decreased bone formation and increased resorption.
Corticosteroid osteoporosis. Due to decreased bone formation and increased resorption.
Heparin-induced osteopenia.
Simple osteoporosis of aging (senile).
Immobilisation. Including weightless space flight.
Deficiency of dietary calcium, protein or ascorbic acid.
Malabsorption syndrome. Due to protein and calcium deficiency.
Idiopathic juvenile osteoporosis.
Idiopathic adult osteoporosis.
Osteogenesis imperfecta. Rare hereditary syndrome of collagen metabolism.

Clinical features

Considerable bone loss necessary before symptoms apparent. Progressive back pain, kyphosis and vertebral collapse (with or without spinal nerve compression). Other pathological fractures including metatarsals, femoral neck and lower end of radius. Other clinical features related to underlying disease process (see relevant section). Juvenile osteoporosis represents a self-limiting process with pain and deformity in childhood spontaneously resolving after puberty. Osteogenesis imperfecta associated with multiple fractures in childhood and blue sclerae.

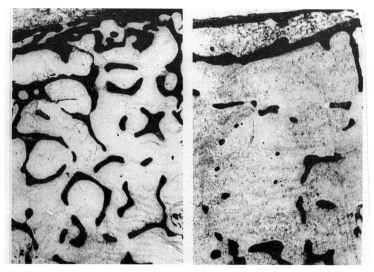

Fig. 135 Bone biopsies of normal (left) and osteoporotic (right) bone taken from iliac crest: note reduction in trabeculae.

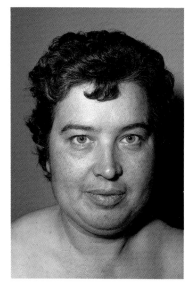

Fig. 136 Patient with Cushing's disease presenting only with back pain.

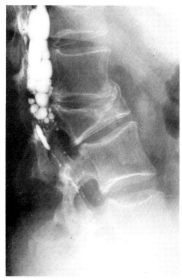

Fig. 137 Same patient: vertebral collapse. Generalised osteoporosis: contrast medium from myelogram.

Diagnosis

Differential diagnosis of cause requires careful consideration of possible underlying factors. No biochemical abnormality attributable to osteoporosis alone—serum calcium, phosphate, alkaline phosphatase normal. Radiology shows decreased bone density in skull, spine, and long bones with narrowed cortical width, especially apparent in metacarpals. Density quantifiable by photon absorptiometry or quantitative CT scanning techniques. Bone biopsy confirms decreased bone mass with normal thickness osteoid seams.

Prevention

Premature menopause (natural or operative) justifies oestrogen replacement until age 55. Maintained activity pattern in all elderly subjects essential. Alternate day corticosteroid therapy for anti-inflammatory medication. Possible protective effect of life-long positive calcium balance.

Treatment

Only exercise (swimming, walking) has possible benefit in increasing bone mass. Calcium supplements with sodium fluoride, oestrogen (androgen in males) and probably vitamin D may prevent further deterioration in early osteoporosis.

Complications

Untreated. Progressive loss of height, deformity and fracture.
Treated. Complications of oestrogen therapy (thromboembolism: increased risk of uterine malignancy). Fluorosis with fluoride therapy, hypercalcaemia with vitamin D overdosage.

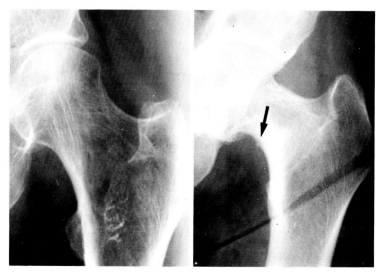

Fig. 138 Two femoral heads showing osteoporosis: reduction in trabecular markings. Patient on right had coexistent osteomalacia due to malabsorption syndrome: note pseudo-fracture (arrow).

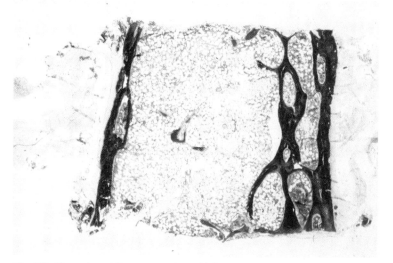

Fig. 139 Hyperthyroidism presenting with bone pain. Bone biopsy shows osteoporosis: major reduction in (dark blue) trabeculae.

34 | Hypoparathyroidism

Occurrence

Prevalence of idiopathic disease 1 : 50 000. 1 : 50 in post-thyroidectomy patients.

Aetiology/ Pathogenesis

Iatrogenic. Excision or devascularisation of para-thyroids during neck (especially thyroid) surgery. *Idiopathic.* Autoimmune destruction associated with familial thyrogastric cluster (see pp. 3, 9, 15, 33, 41, 93). Associated with HLA-B8, DR3, DR4.

Clinical features

May be asymptomatic. Hypocalcaemia induces circum-oral and fingertip paraesthesia and carpal or pedal spasm (especially with cuff-induced ischaemia of limb). Overt tetany occurs in some cases. Chronic cases have posterior subcapsular cataract. Impaired growth with poor dentition in children. Rare cases have basal ganglia calcification.

Diagnosis

Hypocalcaemia, hyperphosphataemia and low serum alkaline phosphatase are characteristic. *Pseudo-hypoparathyroidism.* Similar symptoms and biochemistry but patients have defective renal rubular response to parathormone. Associated mental deficiency, round facies, and basal ganglia calcification on lateral skull radiology. *Osteomalacia.* (See p. 83). Low serum calcium and phosphate, usually with elevated alkaline phosphatase.
Other causes of hypocalcaemia, including low serum binding proteins, may require exclusion.

Treatment

Alpha-calcidol (1α-hydroxy-vitamin D) 0.5−1.0 μg daily with or without calcium supplements are necessary to normalise serum calcium and phosphate. Alternatively calcitriol.

Complications

Untreated. Chronic neuromuscular irritability and cardiac arrhythmias with ectopic calcification in basal ganglia and cerebral cortex resulting in extra pyramidal neurological signs and epilepsy. *Treated.* Overdose with vitamin D analogues induces hypercalcaemia, nephrolithiasis, nephrocalcinosis and ultimately chronic glomerular failure.

METABOLIC BONE DISEASE

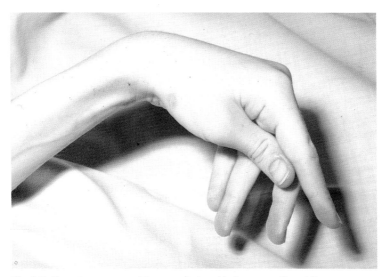

Fig. 140 Spontaneous carpal spasm (tetany) in hypoparathyroidism following total thyroidectomy.

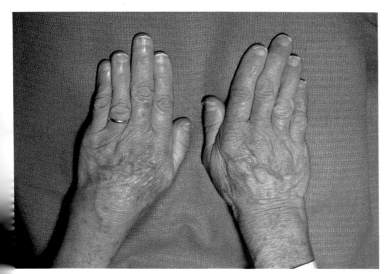

Fig. 141 Hands of patient with pseudohypoparathyroidism: note short 4th metacarpal (brachydactyly) (see also Fig. 114).

Occurrence

Incidence difficult to establish.

Aetiology/ Pathogenesis

Polypeptides from tumours not normally associated with endocrine activity: not all are identical to physiological hormones. Most likely represents derepression of genomes which then become available for DNA transcription. Some as yet unidentified substances may also contribute to tumour cachexia.

Clinical features

Ectopic ACTH. Often oat-cell or C-cell carcinoma (medullary thyroid, thymoma). Rapidly developing Cushing's syndrome with dominant mineralocorticoid effects (oedema, hypertension and hypokalaemia) with weakness dominant.
Ectopic vasopressin. Often oat-cell, but wide range of tumour types. Nausea, vomiting, lethargy and headache leading occasionally to confusion and coma due to cerebral oedema.
Ectopic parathormone. Breast, bronchus, prostate and gastrointestinal tumours. Nausea, vomiting and weakness with later renal failure. Some cases of hypercalcaemia due to osteolytic metastases rather than ectopic hormone secretion.
Ectopic gonadotrophin. Usually tumours of trophoblast (teratoma or choriocarcinoma) resulting in gynaecomastia in males and menstrual irregularity in females.
Ectopic thyrotrophin. Production of alpha subunit of TSH (shared with gonadotrophin) by trophoblast tumours. Biochemical hyperthyroidism more common than overt clinical thyrotoxicosis.
Ectopic erythropoietin. In renal carcinoma, erythropoietin production induces polycythaemia (not strictly an ectopic syndrome). Cerebellar haemangioblastoma may also produce true ectopic erythropoietin.

MISCELLANEOUS

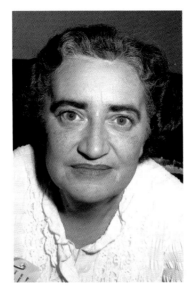

Fig. 142 Ectopic ACTH syndrome due to oat cell carcinoma: control achieved with metyrapone.

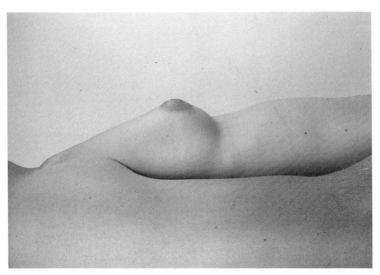

Fig. 143 Sudden evolution of gynaecomastia in male age 51. Ectopic gonadotrophin associated with bronchial carcinoma.

35 | Ectopic Hormone Syndromes (2)

Clinical features

Ectopic growth hormone. Pancreatic and bronchial carcinoma: acromegaly by production of growth hormone releasing factor rather than growth hormone.

Ectopic hypoglycaemia. Rare non-beta cell tumours produce insulin: alternatively excess consumption of glucose by large mesotheliomata or possible inhibition of glycogenolysis.

Diagnosis

Suspect in any case of 'normal' hormone excess. Conversely, in patients with malignancy, ectopic hormone secretion may contribute to the disabling symptoms.

Ectopic ACTH. May be in abnormal (macromolecular) form, or as precursor beta-lipotrophin or beta-endorphin (see p. 37).

Ectopic vasopressin. Identified by hyponatraemia, low serum (<290 mosm/kg) and high urine osmolality.

Ectopic parathormone. Molecular form different to that recognised by standard antibody: serum PTH usually suppressed (see p. 81).

Ectopic gonadotrophin. Elevated beta-hCG levels (see p. 67).

Ectopic thyrotrophin. Usually undetectable serum TSH: beta-hCG almost invariably elevated.

Ectopic erythropoietin. Elevated plasma erythropoietin levels.

Ectopic growth hormone. May present as 'normal' acromegaly (see p. 31).

Ectopic hypoglycaemia. Suppressed plasma insulin by radioimmunoassay.

Treatment

Tumour removal occasionally reverses endocrine syndrome. Ectopic vasopressin syndrome treatable by fluid restriction or demeclocyclin (renal tubular inhibitor of ADH effect). Other syndromes: see pp. 31, 37, 67, 79).

Complications

Those of the underlying syndrome.

MISCELLANEOUS

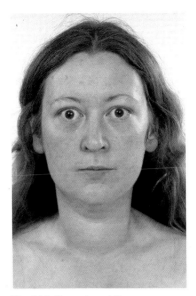

Fig. 144 Hyperthyroidism
associated with choriocarcinoma:
remission following chemotherapy.

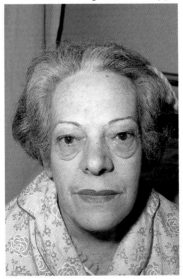

Fig. 145 Acromegaly associated
with carcinoma bronchus:
co-incidence could not be excluded.

36 | Multiple Endocrine Adenomatosis (MEA)

Occurrence

Rare.

Aetiology/ Pathogenesis

Autosomal dominant inheritance (with variable penetrance) in three distinct pluriglandular syndromes. Multiplicity of individual endocrine anomalies both within individuals, or in different members of same kinship. Aetiological mechanism unknown, but in MEA type II and III, common derivation from neural-crest-derived APUD (amine precursor uptake and decarboxylation) cells may be relevant.

Clinical features

MEA type I (Wermer's syndrome). Includes: parathyroid adenoma or hyperplasia (hyperparathyroidism); pancreatic islet adenoma (insulinoma, gastrinoma, somatostatinoma, glucagonoma); pituitary adenoma (functioning or non-functioning); adrenal cortical adenoma (Cushing's syndrome or hyperaldosteronism); carcinoid tumour of small bowel.
MEA type II (Sipple's syndrome). Includes; parathyroid adenoma or hyperplasia (hyperparathyroidism), C-cell tumours (medullary thyroid carcinoma, thymoma) and phaeochromocytoma.
MEA type III Includes: C-cell tumours (as above); adrenal medullary tumour (phaeochromocytoma); multiple cutaneous and mucosal neuromas, neurofibromas and ganglioneuromas (see fig. 12).

Diagnosis

Awareness of other elements of MEA syndromes in any patient presenting with an apparently single element, or with a relevant family history. Individual diagnostic tests detailed in previous sections for specific disorder.

Treatment

As for individual disorders. Screening of first-degree relatives of patients with C-cell tumours by serum calcitonin measurement is controversial.

Complications

Relating to individual disorders.

MISCELLANEOUS

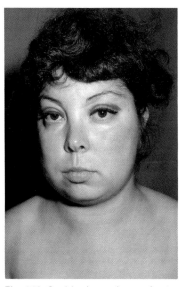

Fig. 146 Cushing's syndrome due to adrenal adenoma. Patient also had hyperparathyroidism: serum calcium 3.1 mmol/1.

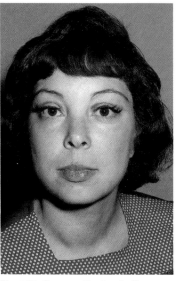

Fig. 147 Same patient as in Figure 146, 6 months after excision of left adrenal adenoma and right lower parathyroid adenoma.

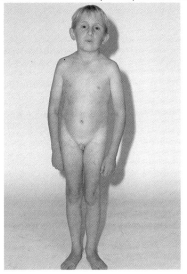

Fig. 148 13-year-old with short stature due to pituitary chromophobe adenoma. Father had similar lesion (age 40).

Multiple Endocrine Deficiency Syndromes (Thyrogastric Cluster)

Occurrence

Common. 1 : 8 subjects with apparently single organ-specific immune lesion either has, or will develop a second lesion, or have an affected first-degree relative.

Aetiology/ Pathogenesis

Linked to abnormality in short arm of chromosome 6: linkage to HLA-B8, DR3, DR4 in most populations. Organ-specific antibodies identifiable for most defined lesions, but relevance to aetiology not always proven.

Type I (insulin-dependent) diabetes mellitus
Hashimoto's disease
Hypothyroidism (juvenile and adult autoimmune)
Graves' disease (hyperthyroidism)
Adrenocortical deficiency (Addison's disease)
Pernicious (Addisonian) anaemia
Vitiligo
Premature ovarian failure
Idiopathic hypoparathyroidism
Systemic and mucocutaneous moniliasis
Hypophysitis (idiopathic hypopituitarism)
Alopecia.
(Idiopathic thrombocytopenic purpura and gluten-sensitive enteropathy may also be members of this syndrome.)

Clinical features

Those of the individual conditions listed (see appropriate section). Premature ovarian failure may occur as early as age 16. Proneness to candida infection (moniliasis) represents a poorly defined immune deficiency.

Diagnosis

Awareness of multiple deficiencies in both individuals and families with one lesion essential. Time of onset of various components may differ by up to 30 years within individuals. Organ-specific antibodies may antedate appearance of clinical syndromes.

Treatment

That of underlying disorder. Premature ovarian failure treated by cyclic oestrogen supplements.

Complications

See individual conditions.

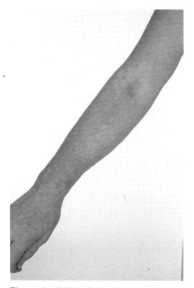

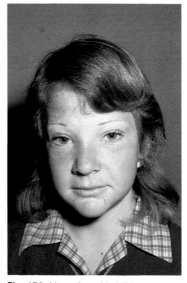

Fig. 149 Vitiligo in patient with Graves' disease. One sister had pernicious anaemia.

Fig. 150 Hypothyroid child presenting with growth failure. Administration of T4 precipitated acute Addison's disease.

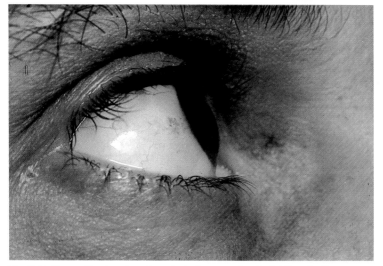

Fig. 151 Generalised and conjunctival pigmentation in Addison's disease. Steroid repletion precipitated acute insulin-dependent diabetes.

Appendix 1: Normal Laboratory Ranges

Blood

Glucose (venous serum): decrease by 1 mmol/l for whole blood	Fasting	< 7 mmol/l
	60 min after 75 g dextrose	< 11 mmol/l
	120 min after 75 g dextrose	< 7 mmol/l
Aldosterone	Ambulant and normal diet (Na^+:100−200 mmol; K^+:50−80 mmol/24 h)	200−800 pmol/l
Cortisol	09.00 h	250−700 nmol/l
	24.00 h	⩽ 200 nmol/l
Corticotrophin	09.00 h	40−120 ng/l
	24.00 h	5−50 ng/l
Follicle-stimulating hormone	Children (pre-pubertal)	< 2.5 U/l
	Adult males	1−7 U/l
	Adult females:	
	Pre-menopausal	1−10 U/l
	Mid-cycle peak	6−25 U/l
	Post-menopausal	30−120 U/l
Luteinising hormone	Male	1.5−10 U/l
	Female:	
	Early follicular	2.5−15 U/l
	Mid-follicular	⩽ 20 U/l
	Mid-cycle peak	25−65 U/l
	Luteal	⩽ 13 U/l
	Post-menopausal	> 25 U/l
17B-Oestradiol	Male	< 175 pmol/l
	Female:	
	Follicular	75−200 pmol/l
	Mid-follicular	350−1500 pmol/l
	Luteal phase	200−1100 pmol/l
	Post-menopausal	< 200 pmol/l
Progesterone	Follicular	⩽ 10.0 nmol/l
	Luteal	20−60 nmol/l
17-Hydroxy-progesterone	Morning sample	⩽ 15 nmol/l
Prolactin		⩽ 800 mU/l
Parathyroid hormone	(C/N terminal antibody)	⩽ 0.73 μg/l
Testosterone	Male	13−30 nmol/l
	Female	0.5−2.5 nmol/l

Sex hormone binding globulin	Male	20–45 nmol DHT/l
	Female	35–100 nmol DHT/l
Insulin	Fasting	$\leqslant$ 20 mU/l
Growth hormone	Resting	$\leqslant$ 10 mU/l
Renin activity	Recumbent: 'Normal' diet (Na^+:100–200 mmol; K^+:50–80 mmol/24 h)	0.5–2.0 pmol/h.ml^{-1}
Thyrotrophin		0.5–3.5 mU/l
Thyroxine		60–160 mmol/l
Free thyroxine		10–25 pmol/l
Tri-iodothyronine		1.4–3.0 nmol/l
25-Hydroxy-cholecalciferol (25-hydroxy vitamin D)		15–100 nmol/l
Vasopressin		1–2 mU/l

Urine (24-h collection)

Aldosterone	'Normal' diet (Na^+: 100–200 mmol; K^+: 50–80 mmol/24 h)	10–25 nmol/l
Free cortisol		100–275 nmol
Total oestrogens	Male	25–85 nmol
	Female:	
	Follicular	25–100 nmol
	Ovulatory peak	140–340 nmol
	Luteal	100–340 nmol
Pregnanetriol	Male	3–6 μmol
Dehydroepian-drosterone	Male	0.35–7 μmol
	Female	0.7–1.75 μmol
Vanillymandelic acid		<40 μmol

Appendix 2: Growth Charts

Growth chart representing the normal range of male development (see p. 73)

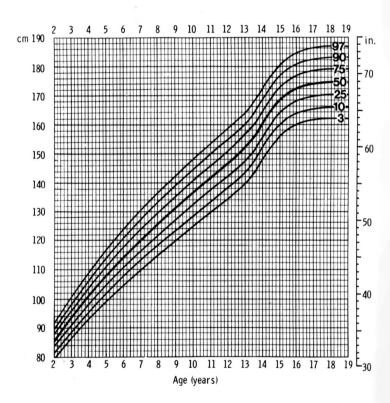

Growth chart representing the normal range of female development (see p. 73)

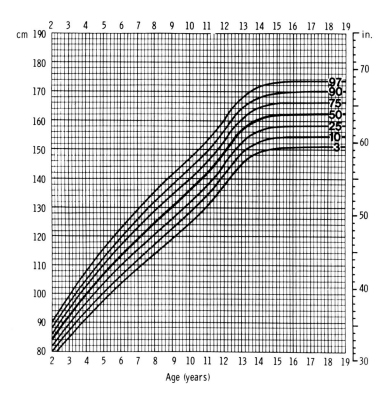

Appendix 3: Adult Desirable Weight

Deviation of 2.5 kg (5 pounds) above or below stated figure represents acceptable limits.

Height (without shoes)		Weight				
		Men			Women	
Feet/Inches	Centimetres	Pounds	Kilograms		Pounds	Kilograms
4/10	147.5	–	–		107	48.5
4/11	150.0	–	–		110	50.0
5/0	152.5	–	–		113	51.5
5/1	155.0	–	–		116	52.5
5/2	157.5	129	58.5		119	54.0
5/3	160.0	133	60.5		122	55.5
5/4	162.5	136	62.0		126	57.0
5/5	165.0	139	63.0		130	59.0
5/6	167.5	143	65.0		135	61.0
5/7	170.0	147	66.5		139	63.0
5/8	172.5	152	69.0		143	65.0
5/9	175.5	156	71.0		147	66.5
5/10	178.0	160	72.5		151	58.5
5/11	180.5	165	75.0		155	70.5
6/0	183.0	170	77.0		–	–
6/1	185.5	175	79.5		–	–
6/2	188.0	180	81.5		–	–
6/3	190.5	185	83.5		–	–
6/4	193.0	190	86.0		–	–

Appendix 4: Abbreviations

ACTH	Adrenocorticotrophic hormone
ADH	Anti-diuretic hormone
AFN	Autonomous hyperfunctioning nodule
AVP	Anginine vasopressin
BR	Background retinopathy
CAH	Congenital adrenal hyperplasia
CRF	Corticotrophin releasing factor
CT	Computerised tomography
DHAS	Dihydroepiandosterone sulphate
DKA	Diabetic ketoacidosis
DNA	Deoxyribonucleic acid
EEG	Electroencephalogram
FSH	Follicle stimulating hormone
GnRH	Gonadotrophin releasing hormone
hCG	Human choriouic gonadotrophin
hGH	Human growth hormone
HLA	Human leukocyte antigen
I^{131}	Radioactive iodine
LH	Luteinising hormone
MEA	Multiple endocrine adenomatosis
MIBG-I^{131}	Meta-iodobenzyl guanidine
MNG	Multinodular goitre
MTG	Multinodular toxic goitre
PR	Proliferative retinopathy
PTH	Parathyroid hormone
SHBG	Sex hormone binding globulin
T4	Thyroxine
T3	Tri-iodothyronine
^{99m}Tc	Technetium
TRH	Thyrotrophin releasing hormone
TSH	Thyroid stimulating hormone
VMA	Vanillylmandelic acid